Essentials of
Nutrition

Essentials of
Nutrition

Sunil Natha Mhaske
MD (Paediatrics)

Professor and Head, Department of Paediatrics
Padmashree Dr Vithalrao Vikhe Patil Medical College
Ahmednagar, Maharashtra

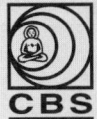

CBS

CBS Publishers & Distributors Pvt Ltd

New Delhi • Bengaluru • Chennai • Kochi • Kolkata • Mumbai
Bhopal • Bhubaneswar • Hyderabad • Jharkhand • Nagpur • Patna • Pune
Uttarakhand • Dhaka (Bangladesh) • Kathmandu (Nepal)

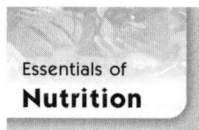

Essentials of
Nutrition

ISBN: 978-81-239-2528-8

Copyright © Author and Publisher

First Edition: 2015
Reprint: 2017, 2020

Published by Satish Kumar Jain and produced by Varun Jain for

CBS Publishers & Distributors Pvt Ltd
4819/XI Prahlad Street, 24 Ansari Road, Daryaganj, New Delhi 110 002, India.
Ph: 23289259, 23266861, 23266867 Website: www.cbspd.com
Fax: 011-23243014 e-mail: delhi@cbspd.com; cbspubs@airtelmail.in.
Corporate Office: 204 FIE, Industrial Area, Patparganj, Delhi 110 092

Ph: 4934 4934 Fax: 4934 4935 e-mail: publishing@cbspd.com; publicity@cbspd.com

Branches

- **Bengaluru:** Seema House 2975, 17th Cross, K.R. Road,
  Banasankari 2nd Stage, Bengaluru 560 070, Karnataka
  Ph: +91-80-26771678/79 Fax: +91-80-26771680 e-mail: bangalore@cbspd.com
- **Chennai:** 7, Subbaraya Street, Shenoy Nagar, Chennai 600 030, Tamil Nadu
  Ph: +91-44-26680620, 26681266 Fax: +91-44-42032115 e-mail: chennai@cbspd.com
- **Kochi:** 68/1534, 35, 36, Power House Road, Opp. KSEB, Kochi 682018, Kerala
  Ph: +91-484-4059061-65 Fax: +91-484-4059065 e-mail: kochi@cbspd.com
- **Kolkata:** 6/B, Ground Floor, Rameswar Shaw Road, Kolkata 700 014, West Bengal
  Ph: +91-33-22891126, 22891127, 22891128 e-mail: kolkata@cbspd.com
- **Mumbai:** 83-C, Dr E Moses Road, Worli, Mumbai 400018, Maharashtra
  Ph: +91-22-24902340/41 Fax: +91-22-24902342 e-mail: mumbai@cbspd.com

Representatives

• Bhopal	0-8319310552	• Bhubaneswar	0-9911037372	• Hyderabad	0-9885175004
• Jharkhand	0-9811541605	• Nagpur	0-9421945513	• Patna	0-9334159340
• Pune	0-9623451994	• Uttarakhand	0-9716462459	• Dhaka (Bangladesh)	01912-003485
• Kathmandu (Nepal)	977-9818742655				

Printed at Mudrak, Noida, UP, India

to

my dietician
and
Rekha Mhaske

Preface

The book *Essentials of Nutrition* has been prepared to reflect the importance of caloric value and dietary importance in day-to-day life and in medical conditions.

Child health is the core of India's development agenda, the root cause of 70% of diseases is malnutrition. To overcome such problem, I have given detail explanation of every food particle used on daily basis in every household and its importance with nutritive value.

I dedicate this book to everyone who is globally impacted by this huge problem and who is fighting back to overcome malnutrition burden from India and all around the world.

I have tried to provide all the important information of nutrition, and request the readers to suggest for improving the same in the future editions.

Sunil Natha Mhaske

Acknowledgements

First of all, I would like to thank Almighty, for bestowing his auspicious blessing and giving me an opportunity to complete this book.

I am deeply grateful to all at CBS Publishers & Distributors, for believing in this book and their unflinching wisdom and kindness.

I would like to thank my pioneers and encouragers, Dr Sujay Vikhe Patil (CEO of Padmashree Dr Vithalrao Vikhe Patil Foundation), Lt. Gen (Retd) Dr B Sadananda (Secretary General of Padmashree Dr Vithalrao Vikhe Patil Foundation), Dr Abhijit Diwate (Deputy Director), Dr DP Joshi (Principal), and Dr AK Pandey (Medical Superintendent).

I extend thanks to my whole backup group, Dr Ramesh Kothari and my postgraduate students Dr Nishad, Dr Pallavi, Dr Mitesh, Dr Vaibhav, Dr Liza, Dr Kanchan and Dr Aditya.

This dream would not have been a reality without support of my wife, Dr Rekha and my kids, Ruchaa and Prabhat.

Sincere thanks to Mr Ramesh Krishnamachari, Regional Manager, from CBS Publishers & Distributors and the entire management for their timely support in bringing out this handbook.

I am open to all for your valuable feedback. Please contact me on *sunilmhask1970@gmail.com*

Sunil Natha Mhaske

Contents

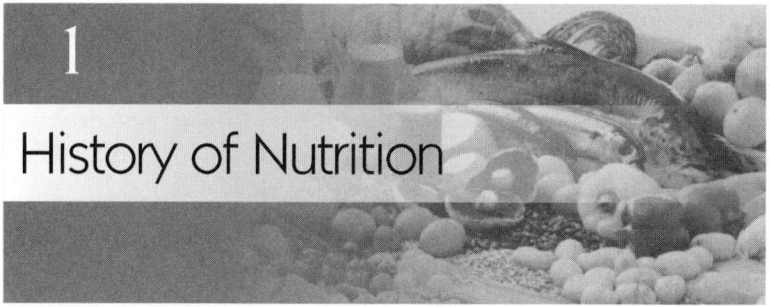

1
History of Nutrition

Introduction

The first record of nutrition goes back to the Book of Daniel in the Bible. In this there is a story mentioned that King of Babylon has captured him and was put on King's table of fine foods and wine but he refused that food and preferred vegetables of which he knew nutritive values and survived on it successfully.

Hippocrates

400 BC: "Father of Medicine"

His famous sentence regarding nutrition is "Let thy food be thy medicine and thy medicine be thy food". He also said, "A wise man should consider that health is the greatest of human blessings."

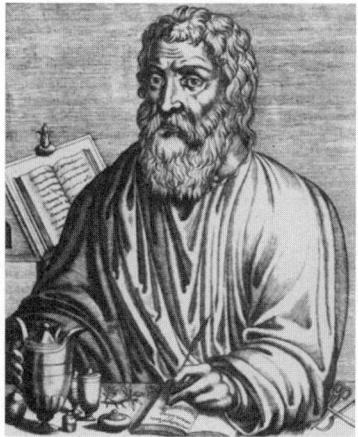

Anaxagoras

475 BC: He stated that food is absorbed by the human body suggesting the existence of nutrients.

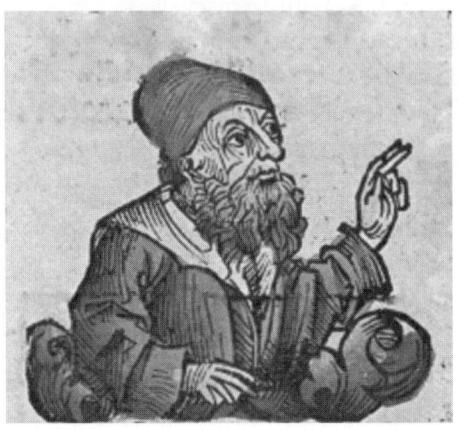

Leonardo da Vinci

1500's: Scientist and artist who compared the process of metabolism in the body to the burning of a candle.

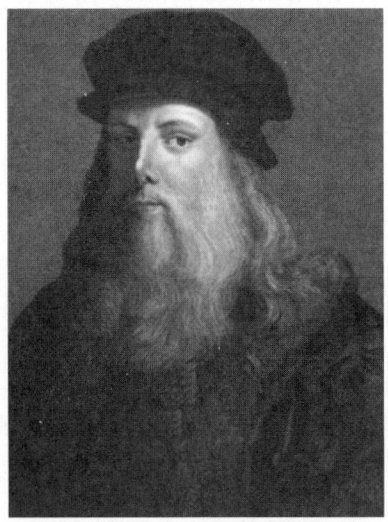

Dr James Lind

He was a British Navy physician who was first to perform the scientific experiment on nutrition. He observed that sailors on long voyages developed scurvy because of consumption of nonperishable foods such as dried meat and breads. There were deficiency of fresh foods. So he used vinegar and limes to sailors and observed absence of scurvy in them.

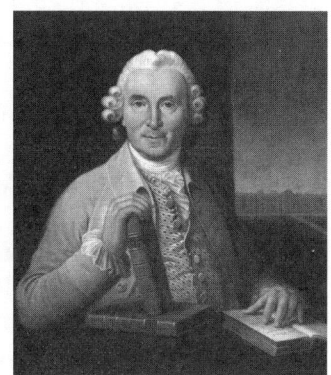

Justus von Liebig

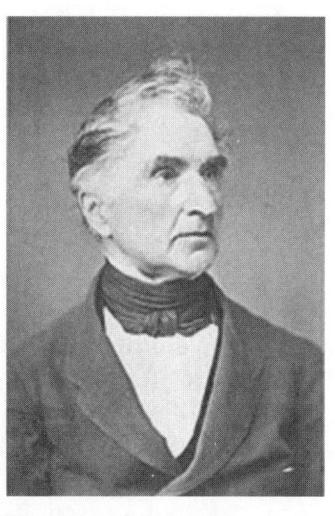

- "Father of Modern Nutrition"
- *Birth*: 12 May 1803
- German chemist
- Eecame a professor at the ℾniversity of Giessen.
- Major contributions to agricultural and biological chemistry
- Established the world's first major school of chemistry
- Greatest chemistry teachers of all time.
- He is considered as the "Father of the Fertilizer Industry".
- Discoverer of nitrogen as an essential plant nutrient.
- Developed a manufacturing process for beef extracts.
- He was elected a member of the Royal Swedish Academy of Sciences in 1837.
- *Death*: 18 April 1873.

Christiaan Eijkman

- *Born*: 11 August 1858, Nijkerk, Netherlands.
- He discovered that food can cure diseases.
- He studied that outer rice bran contains vitamin B_1, also known as thiamine.
- He was appointed as Member of the Royal Netherlands Academy of Arts and Sciences.
- He was Honorary Fellow of the Royal Sanitary Institute in London.
- Government of Indonesia named research center of pathology and bacteriology as Eijkman Institute for Molecular Biology.

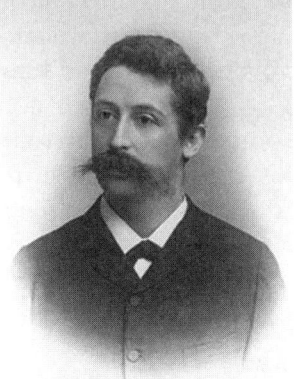

- Dutch physician and professor of physiology whose demonstration that beriberi is caused by poor diet led to the discovery of vitamins. Together with Sir Frederick Hopkins, he received the Nobel Prize for Physiology or Medicine.
- *Died*: 5 November 1930 Utrecht, Netherlands.

EV McCollum

- *Born*: 03 March 1879, Fort Scott, Kansas, US.
- *1912*: He discovered the first fat soluble vitamin, vitamin A also water-soluble vitamin B.
- He also studied that vitamin D prevents rickets.
- He was the first chair and professor in the newly established Department of Chemical Hygiene.
- He published 150 papers at Johns Hopkins.
- In 1946, he wrote two books: *The History of Nutrition* and an autobiography.
- *Died*: November 15, 1967.

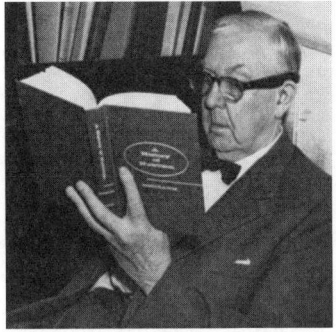

Dr Casmir Funk

- *Born*: February 23, 1884, Warsaw, Russian Empire.
- *1912*: First to coin the term "vitamins" as vital factors in the diet.
- He stated that diseases like rickets, pellagra, sprue and scurvy could be cured by vitamins.
- *Died*: November 20, 1967 New York, United States

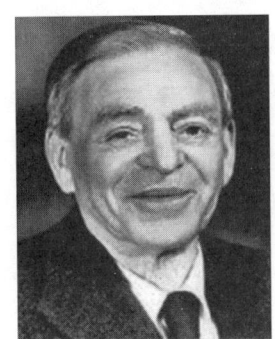

William Rose

(1887–1985)

- He was a professor of biochemistry at University of Illinois.
- He was a pioneer in biochemistry and nutritional science.
- *1930*: He introduced the idea of an essential amino acid into nutrition in both human and rodent diets.
- Also discovered threonine, the essential amino acid that provided a satisfactory diet for rodents when added to other amino acids.

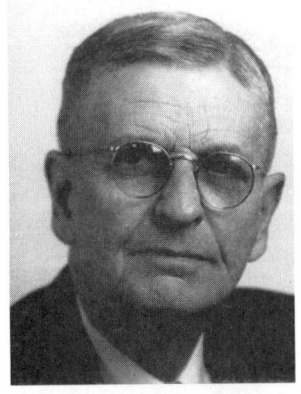

- He also studied lysine, tryptophan, histidine, phenylalanine, leucine, isoleucine, methionine, valine, and arginine in addition to threonine.
- *1936*: He was elected on National Academy of Sciences.
- *1966*: Received the National Medal of Science.
- He was awarded honorary doctor of science degrees by Yale University, the University of Chicago, and the University of Illinois.
- *1952*: He received the Willard Gibbs Medal from the American Chemical Society.
- *1957*: Charles F. Spencer Medal, also of the ACS.

Antoine Lavoisier

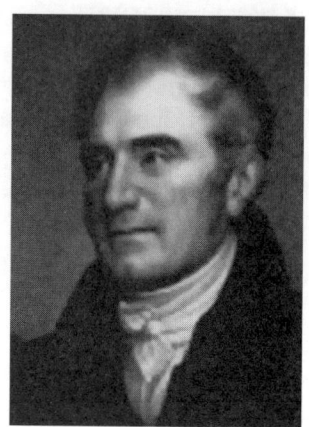

- *Born*: 26 August 1743, Paris, France
- "Father of Nutrition"
- He discovered the actual process by which food is metabolized and role of oxygen in combustion.
- He discovered and named oxygen and hydrogen.
- *1766*: He was awarded a gold medal by the King.
- *Died*: 08 May 1794, Paris, France.
- After his death, a statue of Lavoisier was erected in Paris.

Dr Royal Lee

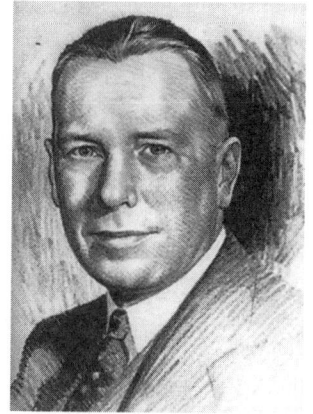

- Father of Holistic Nutrition and *Pioneers of Nutrition.*
- Born on April 7, 1895.
- His theory was whole *nutrient complex is greater than the sum of its parts.*
- *1942*: Received American Association for the Advancement of Science's award.
- *1941*: He founded the Lee Foundation for Nutritional Research, a non-profit education foundation for nutrition.
- He was the best informed person on nutrition in America and perhaps even the world."
- He died in 1967.

Melvin E. Page

- Born in 1894 in Picture Rocks, Pennsylvania.
- Early pioneers in nutritional biochemistry.

- His idea was that eating habit has impact on tooth condition. So eliminate white sugar and white flour from diet.
- He also mentioned that milk is not the perfect food for everyone, whereas eat unlimited quantities of green leafy vegetables.
- He was Fellow of the International College of Applied Nutrition and of the Royal Society of Health (England).

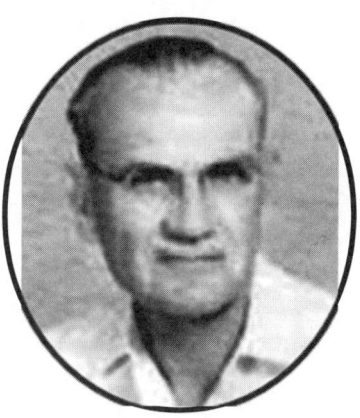

- He published numerous articles on his work in nutrition in such periodicals as the Journal of the American Dental Association, Applied Nutrition, etc.
- He died in 1986.

Weston A Price

(1870–1948)
- He is remembered as "Charles Darwin of Nutrition".
- He studied the relation of causes of dental decay and physical degeneration of teeth.

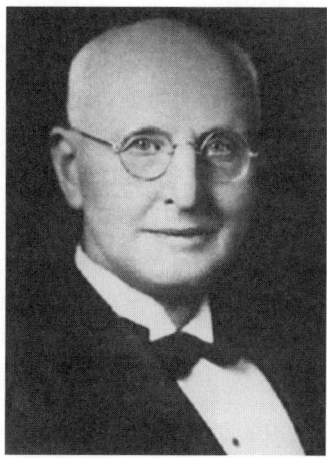

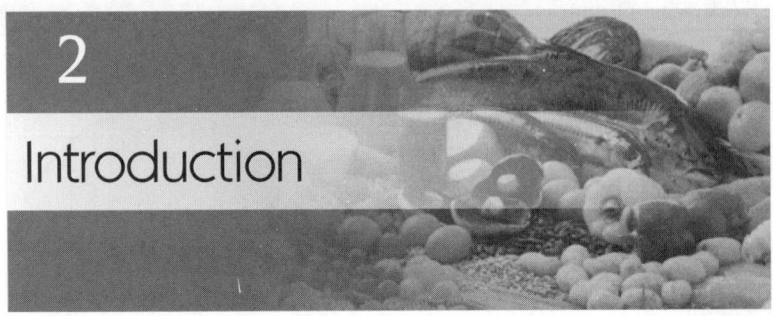

2

Introduction

Definition: The science which deals with the study of foods and its nutrients is called nutrition.

Nutrition has very important role right from *in vitro* fertilization of sperm with an egg, to the birth, up till human growth, maturity, old age, and even death.

Major nutrients in food are: Carbohydrates, fats, dietary fiber, minerals, proteins, vitamins and water.

Carbohydrates

Types: Monosaccharide, disaccharides and polysaccharides.

Dietary fiber is a carbohydrate (a polysaccharide) that is incompletely absorbed in human body.

Fats

Types: Saturated and unsaturated (omega-3 and omega-6 fatty acids).

Proteins

Types: Essential amino acids (cannot be produced in body) and non-essential amino acids (can be produced in human body).

Complete protein contains all the essential amino acids.

Vitamins

Vitamin	Solubility	Recommended dietary allowances
Vitamin A	Fat	900 µg
Vitamin B_1	Water	1.2 mg
Vitamin B_{12}	Water	2.4 µg
Vitamin B_2	Water	1.3 mg
Vitamin B_3	Water	16.0 mg
Vitamin B_5	Water	5.0 mg
Vitamin B_6	Water	1.3–1.7 mg
Vitamin B_7	Water	30.0 µg
Vitamin B_9	Water	400 µg
Vitamin C	Water	90.0 mg
Vitamin D	Fat	10 µg
Vitamin E	Fat	15.0 mg
Vitamin K	Fat	120 µg

Minerals

Macrominerals	Trace minerals
Calcium	Cobalt
Chlorine	Copper
Magnesium	Chromium
Phosphorus	Iodine, zinc
Potassium	Iron, selenium
Sodium	Manganese, vanadium
Sulfur	Molybdenum, nickel

Water: It is an essential nutrient for healthy hydration, which constitutes 60 % of body weight.

From human body water loss is mainly due to:

- Urine excretion (1.5 lit. per day)
- Breathing (0.35 lit. per day)
- Perspiring (0.45 lit. per day)
- Faeces (0.2 lit. per day)

It is advised that drink at least eight ounce glasses or 1.9 liters of water per day.

These food nutrients undergo following processes:

1. Ingestion   2. Digestion
3. Absorption   4. Metabolism
5. Transport   6. Storage
7. Excretion

Energy

Carbohydrates and proteins gives 4 kcal of energy per gram, whereas fats give rise to 9 kcal per gram of food.

Nutrition energy is measured in kilocalories (kcal) or Joule

1 kcal = 4185.8 joules

Balanced diet: A diet which contains adequate amounts of all the necessary nutrients required for healthy growth and activity. Recommended energy from carbohydrates is 45–65% of calories, 10–35% from proteins and 20–35% from fat.

Types of Human Lifestyles

- Sedentary (inactive): Little physical activity in day-to-day functions.
- *Moderately active*: Physical activity equivalent to walking 1.5-to-3 miles per day at 3-to-4 miles per hour, plus normal day-to-day functions.
- *Active physical*: Activity equivalent to walking more than 3 miles per day at 3-to-4 miles per hour, plus normal day-to-day functions.

Gender	Age (years)	Sedentary	Moderately active	Active
Child	2–3	1,000	1,000–1,400	1,000–1,400
Female	4–8	1,200	1,400–1,600	1,400–1,800
	9–13	1,600	1,600–2,000	1,800–2,200
	14–18	1,800	2,000	2,400
	19–30	2,000	2,000–2,200	2,400
	31–50	1,800	2,000	2,200
	51+	1,600	1,800	2,000–2,200

(contd.)

(contd.)

Gender	Age (years)	Sedentary	Moderately active	Active
Male	4–8	1,400	1,400–1,600	1,600–2,000
	9–13	1,800	1,800–2,200	2,000–2,600
	14–18	2,200	2,400–2,800	2,800–3,200
	19–30	2,400	2,600–2,800	3,000
	31–50	2,200	2,400–2,600	2,800–3,000
	51+	2,000	2,200–2,400	2,400–2,800

Nutrition for Children

Nutrition	Food group	Recommended %
Carbohydrates	Cereals and grains	33%
Vitamins and minerals	Various fruits and vegetables	33%
Meat protein	Fish, meat and eggs	12%
Milk proteins	Dairy products	15%
Fat and sugar	Fatty foods, sugary sweets	7%

Food Pyramid

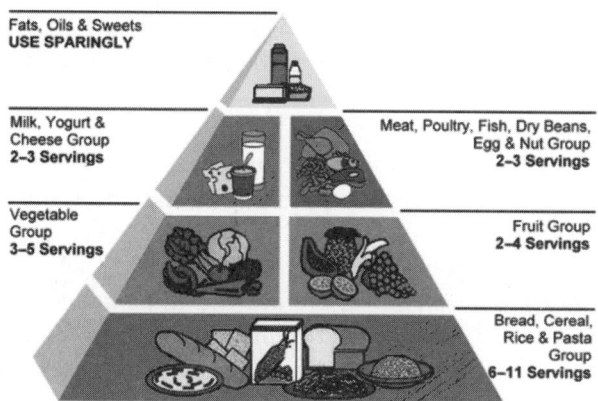

Cautious Foods

- Fried and oily food
- High salt diet
- High sugar diet

World Health Organization Recommendation about Diet

- Increase consumption of plant foods—fruits, vegetables, legumes, whole grains and nuts.
- Limit intake of fats, preferring the healthier unsaturated fats to saturated fats and trans fats.
- Limit the intake of granulated sugar.
- Limit salt and sodium consumption.

Harvard School of Public Health's Recommendations for a Healthy Diet

- Choose good carbohydrates: Whole grains , vegetables, fruits and beans.
- Attention to the protein fish, poultry, nuts, and beans.
- Choose foods containing healthy fats. Plant oils, nuts, and fish are the best choices.
- Choose a fiber-filled diet which includes whole grains, vegetables, and fruits.
- Eat more vegetables and fruits—the more colorful
- Good sources of calcium are collards, bok choy, fortified soy milk, baked beans.
- Water is the best source of liquid. Avoid sugary drinks, and limit intake of juices and milk, coffee, tea, artificially-sweetened drinks.
- Limit salt intake.
- Daily multivitamin and extra vitamin D.

Other than nutrition, frequent physical exercise and maintaining a healthy body weight.

- *Vegetarian diets*: One which excludes meat.
- *Lacto vegetarianism*: A vegetarian diet that includes certain types of dairy products but excludes eggs and foods.
- *Lacto-ovo vegetarianism*: A vegetarian diet that includes eggs and dairy.
- *Vegan diet*: In addition to the requirements of a vegetarian diet, vegans do not eat food produced by animals, such as eggs and dairy products.

Let food be thy medicine and medicine be thy food.

—Hippocrates

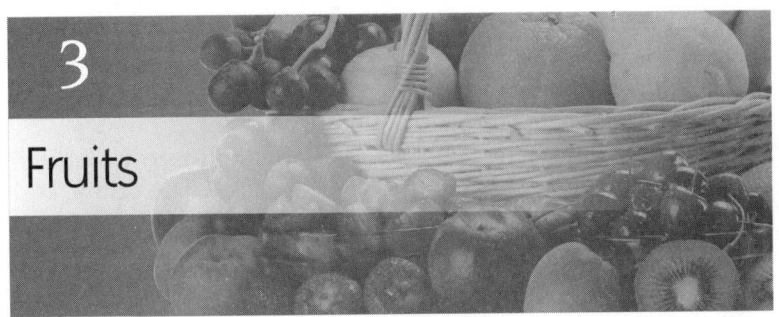

3

Fruits

MANGO

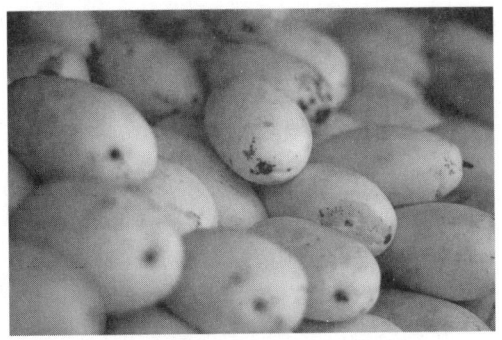

(Per 100 gm)			
Energy	70 kcal	Carbohydrates	17 g
Protein	0.5 g	Fat	0.27 g
Dietary fiber	1.80 g	Sodium	2 mg
Potassium	156 mg	Calcium	10 mg
Copper	0.110 mg	Iron	0.13 mg
Magnesium	9 mg	Zinc	0.04 mg
Vitamin A	765 IU	Vitamin C	27.7 mg
Vitamin E	1.12 mg	Vitamin K	4.2 µg
Thiamin	0.058 mg	Riboflavin	0.057 mg
Pyridoxine	0.134 mg	Pantothenic acid	0.160 mg
Niacin	0.584 mg	Folic acid	14 µg

- Weight gain.
- Prevents acidity and poor digestion.

- Vitamin E boosts up hormonal system function and improves sex life.
- Alleviate asthma.
- Improves concentration and memory power.
- The Glutamine acid in mangoes helps children to have a good memory and keeps the cells active. Antioxidant and antimalignancy property.
- Rich in iron.
- Vitamin A, vitamin E and selenium give protection against heart disease.
- Protects against colon, breast, prostate malignancy and leukemia.
- Boost to the immune system
- Resists infectious agents
- Healthy eye sight prevents night blindness and dry eyes.

BANANA

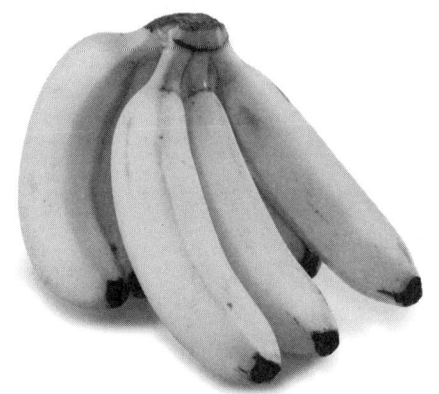

(1 medium size)			
Energy	105 calories	Protein	1.29 grams
Fiber	3.1 grams	Vitamin A	76 IU
Vitamin B_1 (thiamine)	0.037 mg	Vitamin B_2 (riboflavin)	0.086 mg
Niacin	0.785 mg	Vitamin C	10.3 mg
Vitamin E	0.12 mg	Vitamin K	0.6 mcg
Potassium	422 mg	Phosphorus	26 mg
Magnesium	32 mg	Calcium	6 mg
Iron	0.31 mg	Selenium	1.2 mcg
Manganese	0.319 mg	Copper	0.092 mg
Zinc	0.18 mg		

- Pulp is composed of soft, easily digestible flesh with simple sugars like fructose and sucrose that when eaten replenishes energy and revitalizes the body instantly and instant energy.
- Contains health promoting flavonoid poly-phenolic antioxidants such as lutein, zeaxanthin, β and α-carotenes in small amounts—a role in aging and various disease processes.
- Good source of vitamin B_6—a beneficial role for the treatment of neuritis, and anemia.
- Moderate source of vitamin C that resists against infectious contains a good amount of soluble dietary fiber that helps normal bowel movements.
- Adequate levels of copper, magnesium, and manganese. Magnesium is essential for bone manganese as a co-factor for the antioxidant enzyme, superoxide dismutase. Copper is for production of red blood cells.
- Rich source of potassium that helps control heart rate and blood pressure.

ORANGE

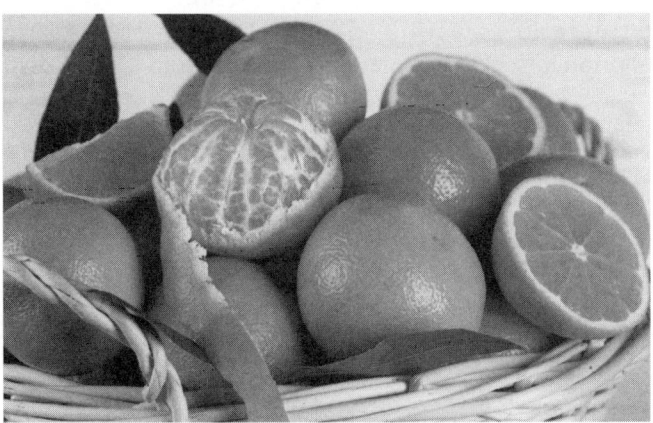

- Low in calories
- No saturated fats or cholesterol
- Rich in dietary fiber, pectin—bulk laxative, reduce blood cholesterol levels.

(One medium)			
Energy	62 calories	Protein	1.23 grams
Fiber	3.1 grams	Potassium	237 mg
Phosphorus	18 mg	Magnesium	13 mg
Calcium	52 mg	Iron	0.13 mg
Copper	0.059 mg	Zinc	0.09 mg
Vitamin A	295 IU	Vitamin B_1	0.114 mg
Vitamin B_2	0.052 mg	Niacin	0.369 mg
Folic acid	39 mcg	Pantothenic acid	0.328 mg
Vitamin B_6	0.079 mg	Vitamin C	69.7 mg
Vitamin E	0.24 mg		

- Excellent source of vitamin C—a powerful natural antioxidant, helps the body develop resistance against infectious.
- Good levels of vitamin A, alpha and beta-carotenes, beta-cryptoxanthin, zeaxanthin and lutein.
- Contains phytochemical—hesperetin, naringin, and naringenin-antioxidant, free radical scavenger, anti-inflammatory and immune system modulator.
- Good source of thiamin, pyridoxine, and folic acid.
- Good amount of potassium and calcium.
- Soluble and insoluble dietary fiber decreases risk of malignancies, arthritis, obesity, and coronary heart diseases.

APPLE

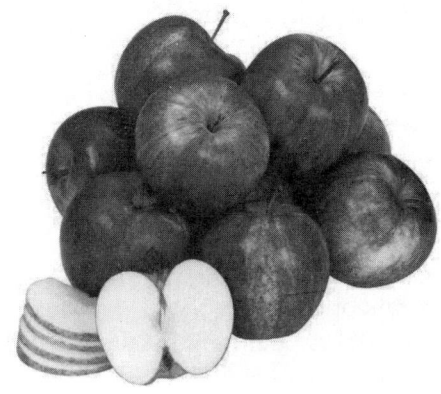

(Per 100 gm)			
Energy	50 kcal	Carbohydrates	13.81 g
Protein	0.26 g	Fat	0.17 g
Cholesterol	0 mg	Fiber	2.40 g
Folic acid	3 µg	Niacin	0.091 mg
Pantothenic	0.061 mg	Pyridoxine acid	0.041 mg
Riboflavin	0.026 mg	Thiamin	0.017 mg
Vitamin A	54 IU	Vitamin C	4.6 mg
Vitamin E	0.18 mg	Vitamin K	2.2 µg
Sodium	1 mg	Potassium	107 mg
Calcium	6 mg	Iron	0.12 mg
Magnesium	5 mg	Phosphorus	11 mg
Zinc	0.04 mg		

- Essential for normal growth and development.
- No saturated fats or cholesterol.
- Rich in dietary fiber, which helps prevent absorption of dietary-LDL or bad cholesterol in the gut.
- Protect from deleterious effects of free radicals.
- Vitamin C helps the body develop resistance against infectious agents and scavenge harmful, pro-inflammatory free radicals from the body.
- Rich in antioxidant phyto-nutrients flavonoids and polyphenolics.
- Rich in potassium, phosphorus, and calcium which helps in controlling heart rate and blood pressure
- Rich in B-complex vitamins which help as co-factors for enzymes in metabolism functions inside the body.

ANJEER

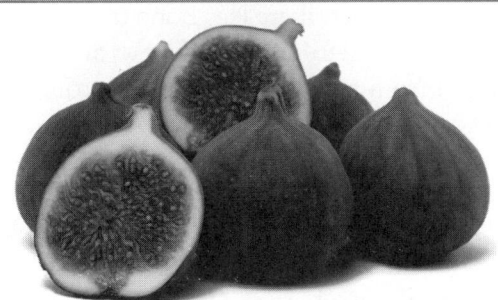

(Quantity—one)			
Energy	47 calories	Protein	0.48 grams
Fiber	1.9 grams	Vitamin K	3 mcg
Potassium	148 mg	Phosphorus	9 mg
Magnesium	11 mg	Calcium	22 mg
Sodium	1 mg	Iron	0.24 mg
Selenium	0.1 mcg	Manganese	0.082 mg
Copper	0.045 mg	Zinc	0.1 mg
Vitamin A	91 IU	Vitamin B_1	0.038 mg
Vitamin B_2	0.032 mg	Niacin	0.256 mg
Folic acid	4 mcg	Pantothenic acid	0.192 mg
Vitamin B_6	0.072 mg	Vitamin C	1.3 mg
Vitamin E	0.07 mg		

- Fig leaves have anti-diabetic properties.
- Rich in fiber which gives protection against breast malignancy.
- Potent bactericide.
- Antifungal property also used to treat warts.
- Contains ficin, which is useful in digestion.
- Keeps healthy bowel function and prevents constipation.
- Gives relief from piles and hemorrhoids.
- Roasted figs are used in the treatment of boils and ulcers in the mouth.
- It reduces the cholesterol level.
- Dried figs contain phenol, omega-3 and omega-6 which reduces the risk of coronary heart disease.
- It reduces body weight.
- If it is taken with milk, it helps in weight gain.
- Rich in calcium which increases bone density
- It is rich in iron—useful in treatment of anemia.
- It gives relief from fatigue and sleep disorders
- Boost up brain power and improves memory.
- It prevents vision loss in older people due to macular degeneration.
- Mashed figs applied on face for acne and pimples.
- Fig soaked in milk overnight and eat them in the morning increases sexual power.

- It is high in potassium but low in sodium, so it controls the blood pressure.

PINEAPPLE

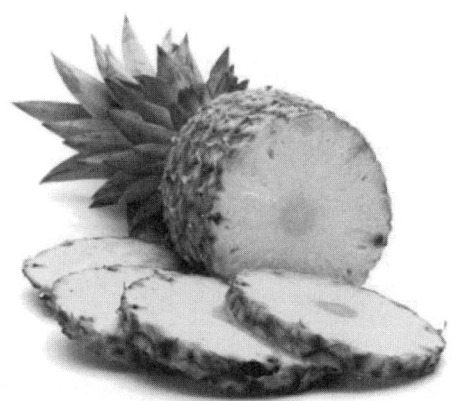

(One cup)			
Energy	82 calories	Protein	0.89 grams
Dietary fiber	2.3 grams	Potassium	180 mg
Phosphorus	13 mg	Magnesium	20 mg
Calcium	21 mg	Sodium	2 mg
Iron	0.48 mg	Selenium	0.2 mcg
Manganese	1.53 mg	Copper	0.181 mg
Zinc	0.2 mg	Vitamin A	96 IU
Vitamin B_1	0.13 mg	Vitamin B_2	0.053 mg
Niacin	0.825 mg	Folic acid	30 mcg
Pantothenic acid	0.351 mg	Vitamin B_6	0.185 mg
Vitamin C	78.9 mg	Vitamin E	0.03 mg
Vitamin K	1.2 mcg		

- No saturated fats or cholesterol.
- Rich source of soluble and insoluble dietary fiber—pectin.
- It contains a proteolytic enzyme—bromelain has anti-inflammatory, anti-clotting and anti-malignancy properties.
- Prevents arthritis, indigestion and worm infestation.
- Excellent source of antioxidant, vitamin C, which protects from scurvy.

- Rich in vitamin A which is required for maintaining healthy mucus membranes, skin and for vision.
- Rich in flavonoids which protects from lung and oral cavity malignancies.
- It contains many minerals like potassium which helps to regulate blood pressure. Copper is a helpful cofactor for red blood cell synthesis. Manganese is a co-factor for the enzyme superoxide dismutase.

WATERMELON

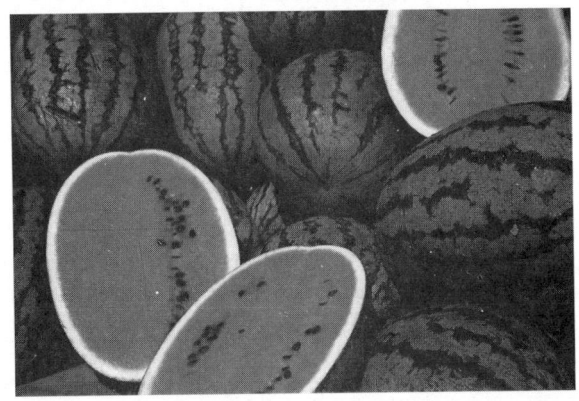

(*1 slice*)			
Energy	86 calories	Protein	1.74 grams
Fiber	1.1 grams	Vitamin A	1627 IU
Vitamin B$_1$	0.094 mg	Vitamin B$_2$	0.06 mg
Niacin	0.509 mg	Folic acid	9 mcg
Pantothenic acid	0.632 mg	Vitamin B$_6$	0.129 mg
Vitamin C	23.2 mg	Vitamin E	0.14 mg
Vitamin K	0.3 mcg	Potassium	320 mg
Phosphorus	31 mg	Magnesium	29 mg
Calcium	20 mg	Sodium	3 mg
Iron	0.69 mg	Selenium	1.1 mcg
Manganese	0.109 mg	Copper	0.12 mg
Zinc	0.29 mg		

- It is a nature's gift for summer thirst.
- Rich in electrolytes and water content.
- Excellent source of vitamin A, which is a powerful natural antioxidant and essential for healthy vision.
- Protect from lung and oral cavity malignancies.
- Good source of potassium which helps in controlling heart rate and blood pressure so giving protection against stroke and coronary heart diseases.
- Rich in antioxidant flavonoids like lycopene, beta-carotene, lutein, zeaxanthin and cryptoxanthin. This gives protection against colon, prostate, breast, endometrial, lung, and pancreatic malignancies.
- Excellent source of carotenoid pigment, lycopene which offers protection to skin from harmful ultraviolet rays.
- It contains good amount of vitamin B_6, thiamin, vitamin C, and manganese. Vitamin C helps the body develop resistance against infectious agents, whereas manganese is a co-factor for the antioxidant enzyme, superoxide dismutase.

PAPAYA

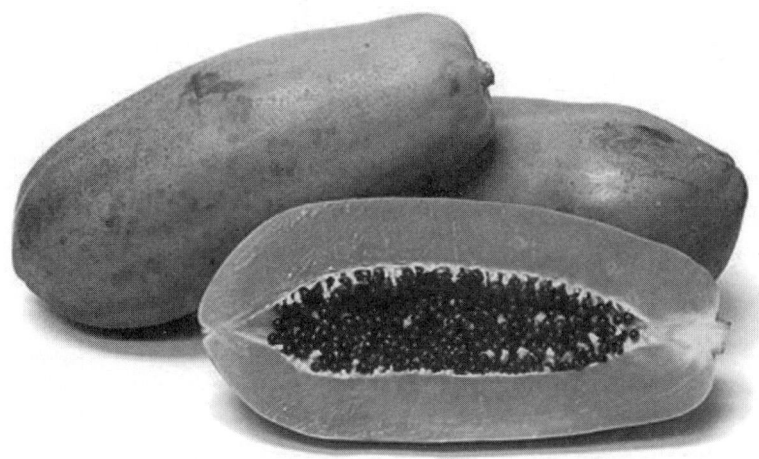

(*One cup*)			
Energy	55 calories	Protein	0.85 gram
Dietary fiber	2.5 grams	Potassium	360 mg
Phosphorus	7 mg	Magnesium	14 mg
Calcium	34 mg	Sodium	4 mg
Iron	0.14 mg	Selenium	0.8 mcg
Zinc	0.1 mg	Manganese	0.015 mg
Copper	0.022 mg	Vitamin A	1532IU
Vitamin B_1	0.038 mg	Vitamin B_2	0.045 mg
Niacin	0.473 mg	Folic acid	53 mcg
Pantothenic acid	0.305 mg	Vitamin B_6	0.027 mg
Vitamin C	86.5 mg	Vitamin E	1.02 mg
Vitamin K	3.6 mcg		

- It has no cholesterol.
- Rich source of phyto-nutrients, minerals, and vitamins.
- Contains soft, easily digestible flesh with a good amount of soluble dietary fiber which avoids constipation.
- Protects the body from lung and oral cavity malignancies.
- Highest vitamin C content which helps to boost up immunity and anti-inflammatory actions.
- Excellent source of vitamin A and flavonoids like β-carotene, lutein, zeaxanthin and cryptoxanthin which plays a role in aging and many disease processes.
- Rich in folic acid, pyridoxine riboflavin, and thiamin which has role in metabolism.
- Contains a good amount of potassium and calcium.
- Papaya seeds are anti-inflammatory, anti-parasitic, analgesic, and used to treat stomachache and ringworm infections.

GUAVA

- Low in calories and fats.
- Rich source of soluble dietary fiber which acts as bulk laxative and relieves constipation.
- Useful in maintaining the integrity of blood vessels, skin, organs, and bones.

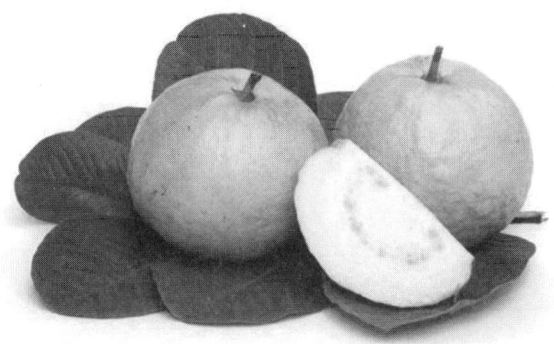

(One cup)			
Energy	112 calories	Protein	4.21 gram
Fiber	8.9 grams	Potassium	688 mg
Phosphorus	66 mg	Magnesium	36 mg
Calcium	30 mg	Sodium	3 mg
Iron	0.43 mg	Selenium	1 mcg
Manganese	0.247 mg	Copper	0.38 mg
Zinc	0.38 mg	Vitamin A	1030 IU
Vitamin B_1	0.111 mg	Vitamin B_2	0.066 mg
Niacin	1.789 mg	Folic acid	81 mcg
Pantothenic acid	0.744 mg	Vitamin B_6	0.181 mg
Vitamin C	376.7 mg	Vitamin E	1.2 mg
Vitamin K	4.3 mcg		

- Lycopene present pink guavas prevents skin damage from UV rays and also offers protection from prostate malignancy.
- Rich source of potassium which helps in controlling heart rate and blood pressure.
- Good source of pantothenic acid, niacin, vitamin B_6, vitamin E, vitamin K, magnesium, copper, and manganese.
- An excellent source of antioxidant vitamin C. More in outer thick rind.
- Good source of vitamin A and flavonoids like beta-carotene, lycopene, lutein and cryptoxanthin. These have antioxidant properties and are essential for optimum health.

STRAWBERRY

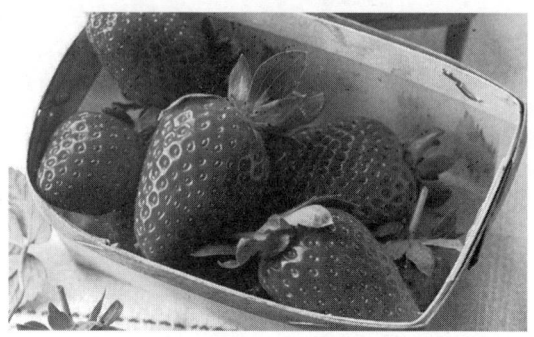

(One cup)			
Energy	46 calories	Protein	0.96 grams
Dietary fiber	2.9 grams	Potassium	220 mg
Phosphorus	35 mg	Magnesium	19 mg
Calcium	23 mg	Sodium	1 mg
Iron	0.59 mg	Selenium	0.6 mcg
Manganese	0.556 mg	Copper	0.069 mg
Zinc	0.2 mg	Vitamin A	17 IU
Vitamin B_1	0.035 mg	Vitamin B_2	0.032 mg
Niacin	0.556 mg	Folic acid	35 mcg
Pantothenic acid	0.18 mg	Vitamin B_6	0.068 mg
Vitamin C	84.7 mg	Vitamin E	0.42 mg
Vitamin K	3.2 mcg		

- Low in calories and fats.
- Contains vitamins A, E and health promoting flavonoid polyphenolic antioxidants such as lutein, zeaxanthin, and beta-carotene in small amount which has a role in aging and various disease processes.
- High amount of phenolic flavonoid phyto-chemicals— anthocyanins and ellagic acid which fights against malignancy, aging, inflammation and neurological diseases.
- Good source of vitamin C which gives protection against infectious agents, inflammation and harmful free radicals.
- Contains good amount of vitamin B_6, niacin, riboflavin, pantothenic acid and folic acid.

- Good amount of potassium, manganese, fluorine, copper, iron and iodine.

AVOCADO

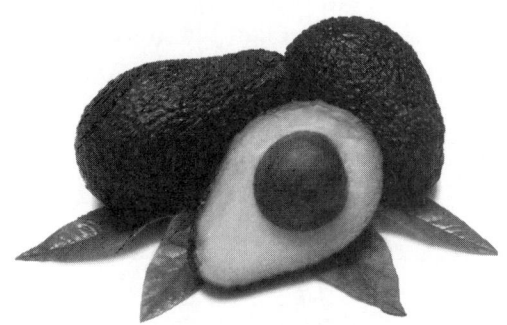

(Per 100 gm)			
Energy	160 kcal	Carbohydrates	8.53 g
Protein	2.0 g	Fat	14.66 g
Dietary fiber	6.7 g	Sodium	7 mg
Potassium	485 mg	Calcium	12 mg
Copper	0.190 mg	Iron	0.55 mg
Magnesium	29 mg	Manganese	0.142 mg
Phosphorus	52 mg	Selenium	0.4 µg
Zinc	0.64 mg	Folic acid	81 µg
Niacin	1.738 mg	Pantothenic acid	1.389 mg
Pyridoxine	0.257 mg	Riboflavin	0.130 mg
Thiamin	0.067 mg	Vitamin A	146 IU
Vitamin C	10 mg	Vitamin E	2.07 mg
Vitamin K	21 µg		

- High-fat content and calories.
- Creamy pulp is a good source of mono-unsaturated fatty acids like oleic and palmitoleic acids as well as omega-6 poly-unsaturated fatty acid linoleic acid. It helps to lower LDL (bad cholesterol) and increase HDL (good-cholesterol) and prevents coronary artery disease and strokes.
- Source of potassium that regulates heart rate and blood pressure.

- Good source of soluble and insoluble dietary fiber which helps to lower blood cholesterol and also prevents constipation.
- Contain high concentration of tannin which is anti-inflammatory, anti-ulcer and antioxidant properties.
- Its flesh contains health promoting flavonoid poly-phenolic antioxidants such as cryptoxanthin, lutein, zeaxanthin, beta and alpha carotenes which play a role in aging and various disease processes.
- Good in vitamins A, E, and K.
- Excellent sources of iron, copper, magnesium, and manganese.

BLACKBERRIES

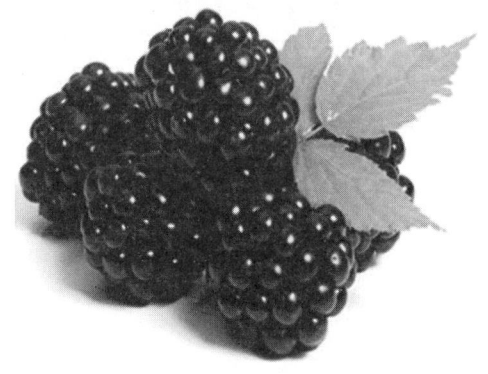

(Per 100 gm)			
Energy	43 kcal	Carbohydrates	9.61 g
Protein	1.39 g	Fat	0.49 g
Cholesterol	0 mg	Dietary fiber	5.3 g
Sodium	1 mg	Potassium	162 mg
Calcium	29 mg	Copper	165 µg
Iron	0.62 mg	Magnesium	20 mg
Manganese	0.646 mg	Selenium	0.4 µg
Zinc	0.53 mg	Folic acid	25 µg
Niacin	0.646 mg	Pantothenic acid	0.276 mg
Pyridoxine	0.030 mg	Thiamin	0.020 IU
Vitamin A	214 IU	Vitamin C	21 mg
Vitamin E	1.17 mg	Vitamin K	19.8 µg

- Low in calories.
- Xylitol is a low-calorie sugar which is absorbed more slowly than glucose inside the gut. That is why it does not cause rapid fluctuations in blood sugar levels.
- Excellent source of vitamin C which has resistance against infectious agents, inflammation, and scavenge harmful free radicals.
- Adequate vitamin A and vitamin E have a role in aging and many disease processes.
- Rich in soluble and insoluble fiber.
- High amount of phenolic flavonoid phytochemicals like asanthocyanins, ellagic acid, tannin, quercetin, gallic acid, cyanidins, pelargonidins, catechins, kaempferol and salicylic acid. These have protective role against malignancy, aging, inflammation, and neurological diseases.
- Good amount of potassium, manganese, copper, and magnesium.
- Good amount of pyridoxine, niacin, pantothenic acid, riboflavin, and folic acid.

BLACKCURRANTS

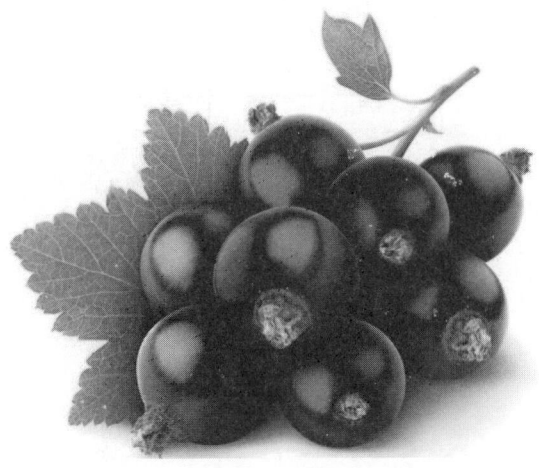

(Per 100 gm)			
Energy	63 kcal	Carbohydrates	15.38 g
Protein	1.4 g	Fat	0.41 g
Cholesterol	0 mg	Dietary fiber	4.3 g
Sodium	2 mg	Potassium	322 mg
Calcium	55 mg	Copper	0.086 mg
Iron	1.54 mg	Magnesium	24 mg
Manganese	0.256 mg	Phosphorus	59 mg
Zinc	0.27 mg	Folic acid	8 µg
Niacin	0.300 mg	Pantothenic acid	0.398 mg
Pyridoxine	0.066 mg	Riboflavin	0.050 mg
Thiamin	0.050 mg	Vitamin A	230 IU
Vitamin C	181 mg		

- Very good in vitamin A and flavonoid anti-oxidants such as beta-carotene, zeaxanthin and cryptoxanthin levels.
- Rich in pantothenic acid, pyridoxine and thiamin.
- Good amount of iron, copper, calcium, phosphorus, manganese, magnesium, and potassium. These are very essential for body metabolism. High amount of phenolic flavonoid phytochemicals—anthocyanins. These protect against malignancy, aging, inflammation, and neurological diseases.
- Excellent source of antioxidant vitamin C which gives immunity against infectious agents and scavenge harmful oxygen-free radicals from the body.

BLUEBERRIES

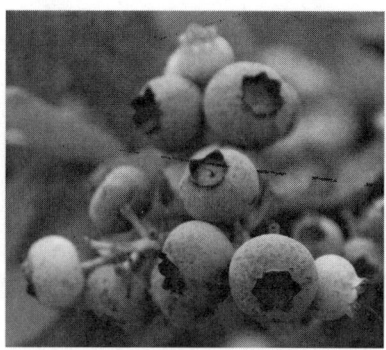

(Per 100 gm)			
Energy	57 kcal	Carbohydrates	14.49 g
Protein	0.74 g	Fat	0.33 g
Cholesterol	0 mg	Dietary fiber	2.4 g
Sodium	1 mg	Potassium	77 mg
Calcium	6 mg	Iron	0.28 mg
Magnesium	6 mg	Manganese	0.336 mg
Zinc	0.16 mg	Folic acid	6 µg
Niacin	0.418 mg	Pantothenic acid	0.124 mg
Pyridoxine	0.052 mg	Riboflavin	0.041 mg
Vitamin A	54 IU	Vitamin C	9.7 mg
Vitamin E	0.57 mg	Vitamin K	19.3 µg

- Very low in calories.
- Highest anti-oxidant properties.
- phyto-chemicals protect the human body against malignancies, aging, degenerative diseases, and infections.
- It lowers the blood sugar levels and controls blood-glucose levels in type-2 diabetes mellitus patients.
- Very good amount of vitamin B_6, niacin, riboflavin, pantothenic acid and folic acid.
- Good amount of potassium, manganese, copper, iron and zinc. Potassium helps controlling heart rate and blood pressure. Manganese acts as a co-factor for the antioxidant enzyme, superoxide dismutase. Copper is required for the production of red blood cells. Iron is required for red blood cell formation.

BOYSENBERRIES

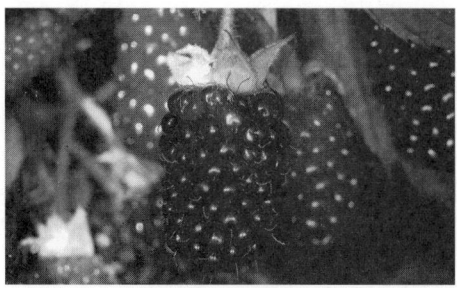

(One cup)					
Energy	66 calories	Protein	1.45 grams	Fiber	7 grams

BREADFRUIT

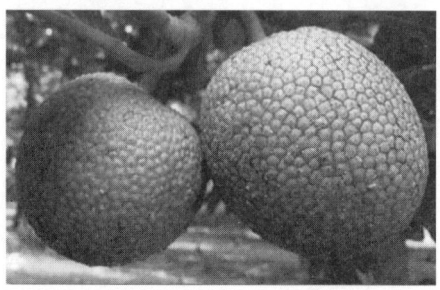

(One cup)					
Energy	227 calories	Protein	2.35 grams	Fiber	10.8 grams

CANTALOUPE (Musk Melon)

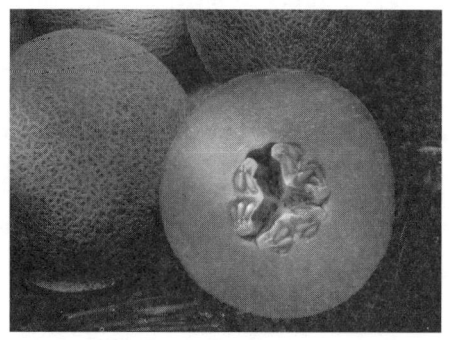

(Per 100 gm)			
Energy	34 kcal	Carbohydrates	8.6 g
Protein	0.84 g	Fat	0.19 g
Cholesterol	0 mg	Dietary fiber	0.9 g
Sodium	1 mg	Potassium	267 mg
Calcium	9 mg	Copper	41 µg
Iron	0.21 mg	Magnesium	12 mg
Manganese	0.041 mg	Zinc	0.18 mg
Folic acid	21 µg	Niacin	0.734 mg
Pantothenic acid	0.105 mg	Pyridoxine	0.072 mg
Riboflavin	0.026 mg	Thiamin	0.017 mg
Vitamin A	3382 IU	Vitamin C	36.7 mg
Vitamin E	0.05 mg	Vitamin K	2.5 mcg

- Have rich flavor
- Very low in calories and fats.
- Excellent source of vitamin A which is a powerful antioxidant having role in vision and protection from lung and oral cavity malignancies.
- Rich in antioxidant flavonoids such as beta carotene, lutein, zeaxanthin and cryptoxanthin. They give protection against colon, prostate, breast, endometrial, lung, and pancreatic malignancies.
- Contains zeaxanthin—dietary carotenoid gives protection to the eyes from age-related macular degeneration.
- Moderate source of potassium which controls heart rate and blood pressure which ultimately gives protection against stroke, and coronary heart diseases.
- Moderate quantity of niacin, pantothenic acid, vitamin C, and manganese.

CHERRIES

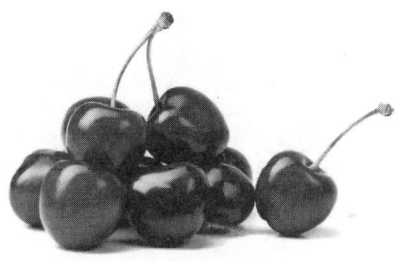

(Per 100 gm)			
Energy	63 cal	Carbohydrates	16.1 g
Protein	1.06 g	Fat	0.2 g
Cholesterol	0 g	Dietary fiber	2.1 g
Folic acid	4 µg	Niacin	0.154 mg
Pantothenic acid	0.199 mg	Pyridoxine	0.049 mg
Riboflavin	0.033 mg	Thiamin	0.027 mg
Vitamin C	7 mg	Vitamin A	640 IU
Vitamin E	0.07 mg	Vitamin K	2.1 µg
Sodium	0 mg	Potassium	222 mg
Calcium	13 mg	Copper	0.060 mg
Iron	0.36 mg	Magnesium	11 mg
Manganese	0.070 mg	Phosphorus	21 mg
Zinc	0.07 mg		

- Very low calorie fruits.
- Pigment rich fruits—polyphenolic flavonoid as anthocyanin glycosides which is a powerful antioxidant.
- It has anti-inflammatory properties by blocking the actions of cyclooxygenase-1, and 2 enzymes. This is useful in diseases like gout arthritis, and sports injuries.
- It gives protection against malignancies, aging, neurological diseases and pre-diabetes condition.
- Rich in stable anti-oxidant melatonin which crosses the blood–brain barrier and decreases irritability, neurosis, insomnia and headache.
- Also source of zinc, iron, potassium, manganese and copper.
- Have a major role against aging, malignancies and many diseases.
- High levels of vitamin C.

DATES

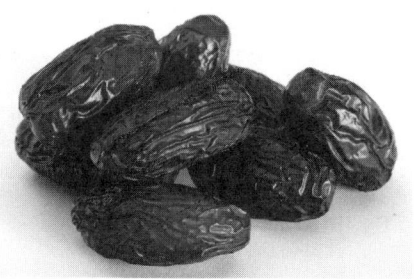

(Per 100 gm)			
Energy	277 kcal	Carbohydrates	74.97 g
Protein	1.81 g	Fat	0.15 g
Cholesterol	0 mg	Dietary fiber	6.7 g
Sodium	1 mg	Potassium	696 mg
Calcium	64 mg	Copper	0.362 mg
Iron	0.90 mg	Magnesium	54 mg
Manganese	0.296 mg	Phosphorus	62 mg
Zinc	0.44 mg	Folic acid	15 µg
Niacin	1.610 mg	Pantothenic acid	0.805 mg
Pyridoxine	0.249 mg	Riboflavin	0.060 mg
Thiamin	0.050 mg	Vitamin A	149 IU
Vitamin C	0 mg	Vitamin K	2.7 µg

- Delicious, easily digestible flesh.
- Contains simple sugars—fructose and dextrose.
- It replenishes energy and revitalize body instantly.
- Religiously used to break the fast during Ramadan month.
- Rich in dietary fiber, which prevents LDL cholesterol absorption in the gut.
- Fiber content is high which acts as a bulk laxative useful in constipation and reducing risk of colon malignancy.
- Very good in potassium which controls heart rate and blood pressure, ultimately offers protection against coronary heart diseases.
- Rich in calcium, manganese, copper, and magnesium.
- Good amount of pyridoxine , niacin, pantothenic acid, and riboflavin.
- Contain flavonoid polyphenolic antioxidants—tannins which is anti-infective, anti-inflammatory and anti-hemorrhagic.
- It contains a dietary carotenoid zeaxanthin which is absorbed into the retinal macula. It gives protection against age-related macular degeneration.
- It contains antioxidant flavonoids such as β-carotene, lutein, and zeaxanthin which gives protection against colon, prostate, breast, endometrial, lung and pancreatic malignancies.
- They are moderate sources of vitamin A which is essential for vision.
- Excellent source of iron which helps in hemoglobin function and oxygen-carrying capacity of the red blood cells.

KIWI

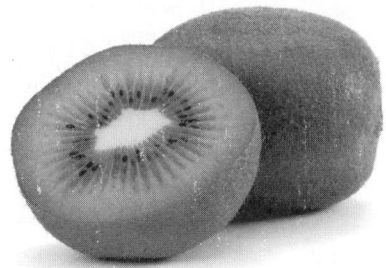

(Per 100 gm)			
Energy	61 kcal	Carbohydrates	14.66 g
Protein	1 g	Fat	0.52 g
Cholesterol	0 mg	Dietary fiber	3 g
Sodium	3 mg	Potassium	312 mg
Calcium	34 mg	Copper	0.130 mg
Iron	0.31 mg	Magnesium	17 mg
Manganese	0.098 mg	Zinc	0.14 mg
Folic acid	25 µg	Niacin	0.341 mg
Riboflavin	0.025 mg	Thiamin	0.027 mg
Vitamin A	87 IU	Vitamin C	92.7 mg
Vitamin E	1.46 mg	Vitamin K	40.3 µg

- Very rich source of soluble dietary fiber—good bulk laxative. It protects the colon mucous membrane by decreasing exposure time to toxins as well as binding to malignancy causing chemicals in the colon.
- Excellent source of antioxidant vitamin C resistance against infectious agents and scavenge harmful free radicals.
- Rich source of potassium help regulate heart rate and blood pressure by countering malefic effects of sodium.
- Good amount of manganese, iron and magneium.
- Very good in vitamin A, vitamin E, vitamin K and flavonoid antioxidants such as beta-carotene, lutein and xanthin.
- Excellent source of omega-3 fatty acids. It reduces the risk of coronary heart disease, stroke, and help prevent the development of ADHD, autism, and other developmental disorders in children.
- Vitamin K has a potential role in the increase of bone mass by promoting osteotrophic activity in the bone. It also has established role in Alzheimer's disease patients by limiting neuronal damage in the brain.
- Functions as blood thinner function similar to aspirin; thus, it helps prevent clot formation inside the blood vessels and protects from stroke and heart attack risk.

LYCHEE

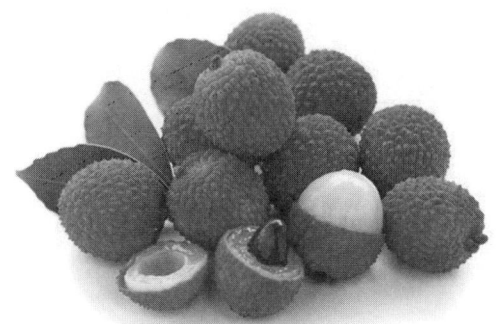

	(Per 100 gm)		
Energy	66 kcal	Carbohydrates	16.53 g
Protein	0.83 g	Fat	0.44 g
Cholesterol	0 mg	Dietary fiber	1.3 g
Sodium	1 mg	Potassium	171 mg
Calcium	5 mg	Copper	0.148 mg
Iron	0.31 mg	Magnesium	10 mg
Manganese	0.055 mg	Phosphorus	31 mg
Selenium	0.6 µg	Zinc	0.07 mg
Folic acid	14 µg	Niacin	0.603 mg
Choline	7.1 mg	Pyridoxine	0.100 mg
Riboflavin	0.065 mg	Thiamin	0.011 mg
Vitamin A	0 mg	Vitamin C	71.5 mg
Vitamin E	0.07 mg	Vitamin K	0.4 µg

- No saturated fats or cholesterol.
- Oligonol, a low molecular weight polyphenol is present abundantly in this fruit. This has an antioxidant and anti-influenza virus actions.
- Rich in potassium and copper. Potassium controls heart rate and blood pressure, whereas copper is required in the production of red blood cells.
- This also helps to reduce weight and protect skin from harmful UV rays.
- Excellent source of vitamin C.
- Good source of thiamin, niacin, and folic acid.

CHINESE PEAR

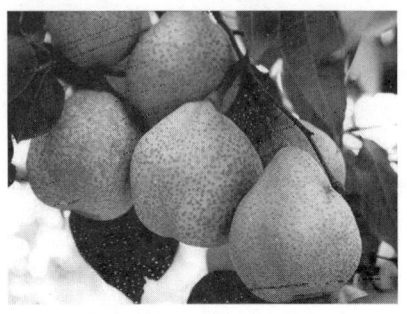

(One fruit)					
Energy	116 calories	Protein	1.38 grams	Fiber	9.9 grams

GRAPES

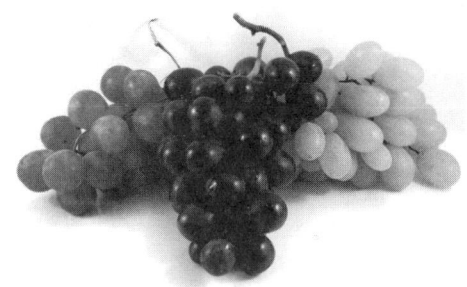

(Per 100 gm)			
Energy	69 kcal	Carbohydrates	18 g
Protein	0.72 g	Fat	0.16 g
Cholesterol	0 mg	Dietary fiber	0.9 g
Sodium	0%	Potassium	191 m
Minerals		Calcium	10 mg
Copper	0.127 mg	Iron	0.36 mg
Magnesium	7 mg	Manganese	0.071 mg
Zinc	0.07 mg	Folic acid	2 µg
Niacin	0.188 mg	Pantothenic acid	0.050 mg
Pyridoxine	0.086 mg	Riboflavin	0.070 mg
Thiamin	0.069 mg	Vitamin A	66 IU
Vitamin C	10.8 mg	Vitamin E	0.19 mg
Vitamin K	14.6 µg		

- Very low in calories.

- It is rich in polyphenolics photochemical—resveratrol which is an antioxidant having role in prevention of colon and prostate malignancies, coronary heart disease, degenerative nerve disease and Alzheimer's disease.

- Rich source of micronutrient like copper, iron and manganese. Copper and manganese are an essential co-factor of antioxidant enzyme, superoxide dismutase.

- Resveratrol also reduces risk of stroke through decreased activity of angiotensin and production of the vasodilator—nitric oxide.

- Another polyphenolics antioxidants present in the red grapes is the anthocyanins which have an anti-allergic, anti-inflammatory, anti-microbial, as well as anti-malignancy property.

- Catechins, a type of flavonoids found in the white and green types have health-protective functions.

- Good source of vitamins C, A, K, pyridoxine, riboflavin and thiamin.

GRAPEFRUIT

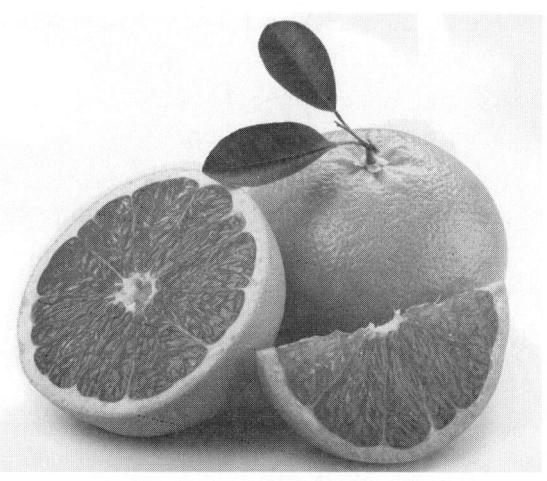

(*Per 100 gm*)			
Energy	42 kcal	Carbohydrates	10.7 g
Protein	0.77 g	Fat	0.14 g
Cholesterol	0 mg	Dietary fiber	1.70 g
Sodium	0 mg	Potassium	135 mg
Calcium	22 mg	Copper	0.032 mg
Iron	0.08 mg	Magnesium	9 mg
Manganese	0.022 mg	Phosphorus	18 mg
Selenium	0.1 µg	Zinc	0.07 mg
Folic acid	13 µg	Niacin	0.204 mg
Pantothenic acid	0.262 mg	Pyridoxine	0.053 mg
Riboflavin	0.031 mg	Thiamin	0.043 mg
Vitamin A	1150 IU	Vitamin C	31.2 mg
Vitamin E	0.13 mg	Vitamin K	0 µg
Lycopene	1419 µg		

- Very low in calories.
- Rich in dietary insoluble fiber pectin which is a bulk laxative helps in constipation and colon malignancy.
- Pectin also reduces blood cholesterol levels by decreasing re-absorption of cholesterol binding bile acids in the colon.
- Good source of vitamin A and flavonoid antioxidants such as naringenin, and naringin.
- Moderate source of lycopene, beta-carotene, xanthin and lutein which are essential for vision.
- Red grapefruits contain lycopene which protects skin from UV rays and protection against prostate malignancy.
- Rich in folic acid, riboflavin, pyridoxine, and thiamin, iron, calcium, copper, and phosphorus.
- Protect from lung and oral cavity malignancies.
- Good source of antioxidant vitamin C.
- Rich in potassium which helps in controlling heart rate and blood pressure.

PLUM

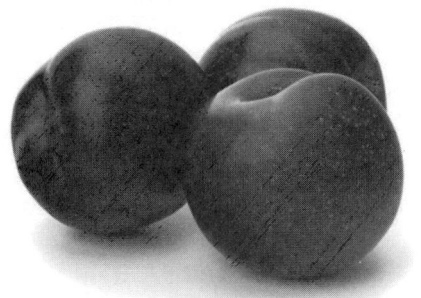

(*One cup*)					
Energy	76 calories	Protein	1.15 grams	Fiber	2.3 grams

STAR FRUIT (Carambola)

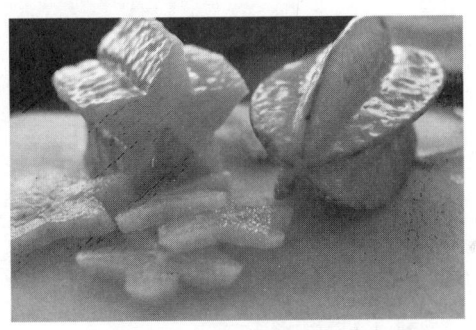

(*Per 100 gm*)			
Energy	31 kcal	Carbohydrates	6.73 g
Protein	1.04 g	Fat	0.33 g
Cholesterol	0 mg	Dietary fiber	2.80 g
Sodium	2 mg	Potassium	133 mg
Calcium	3 mg	Iron	0.08 mg
Magnesium	10 mg	Phosphorus	12 mg
Folic acid	12 µg	Niacin	0.367 mg
Pyridoxine	0.017 mg	Riboflavin	0.016 mg
Thiamin	0.014 mg	Vitamin A	61 IU
Vitamin C	34.4 mg	Vitamin E	0.15 mg
Vitamin K	0 µg		

- Low calorie exotic fruits.
- Peel contains a good amount of dietary fiber which prevents absorption of dietary LDL cholesterol in the gut, also protects the mucous membrane of the colon from malignancy-causing chemicals in the colon.
- Rich in antioxidant phyto-nutrients polyphenolic flavonoids.
- Good source of folic acid, riboflavin, and pyridoxine.
- Also have small amount of potassium, phosphorus, zinc and iron.
- Good amount of vitamin C which fights against infectious agents and scavenge harmful, pro-inflammatory free radicals from the body.

JAMUN—THE INDIAN BLACKBERRIES

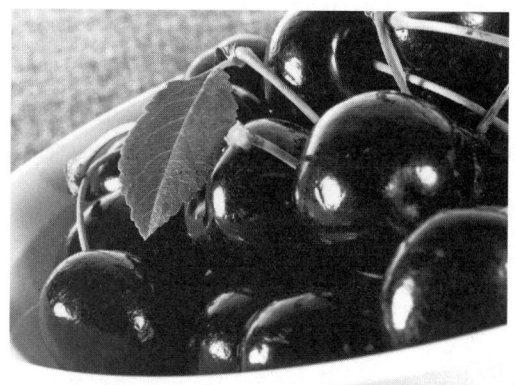

(Per 100 gm)			
Energy	60 kcal	Carbohydrates	15.56 g
Fat	0.23 g	Protein	0.72 g
Water	83.13 g	Vitamin A	3 IU
Thiamine	0.006 mg	Riboflavin	0.012 mg
Niacin	0.260 mg	Pantothenic acid	0.160 mg
Vitamin B_6	0.038 mg	Vitamin C	14.3 mg
Calcium	19 mg	Iron	0.19 mg
Magnesium	15 mg	Phosphorus	17 mg
Potassium	79 mg	Sodium	14 mg

- It is liver protective.
- Fruit has anti-malignancy esp. during chemotherapy and radiotherapy.
- Treatment of diarrhea, dysentery and dyspepsia.
- Useful in ringworm treatment.
- Low calories.
- Rich in carbohydrates and proteins.
- Glucose and fructose are the principal sugars with no sucrose.
- Good source of iron.
- Excellent source of vitamin C.
- Small amount of calcium.
- Rich source of folic acid.
- Good quantity of vitamin B complex, magnesium, potassium, fiber, carotene and phytochemicals (anti-oxidants).
- Stem and bark contains tannin, gallic acid, resin, phytosterols.
- Bark is used as de-worming.
- Herbal medicine in urinary disorders.
- Fruit is used in ayurvedic, unani and chinese medicine.
- Fruit acts as a dieuretic.
- Bark is used in ulcerative colitis, spongy gums and stomatitis.
- Prevents excessive urination or sweating.
- Good source of polyphenolics which helps in prevention of malignancy, heart diseases, diabetes and arthritis.
- Seed contains the glycoside, jamboline, gallic acid and essential oils.
- Leaves contain essential oils.
- Flower contains terpenoids.
- Fruits, leaves, seeds and bark decreases the blood sugar level.
- Bark and leaves control high blood pressure.

COCONUT

- Complete food.
- Rich in calories, vitamins, and minerals.

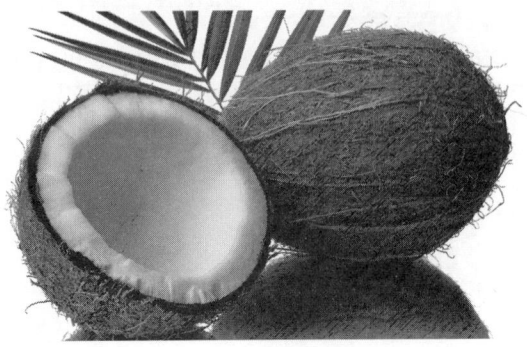

(Per 100 gm)			
Energy	354 kcal	Carbohydrates	24.23
Sugars	6.23	Fiber	9
Fat	33.49	Protein	3.33 g
Calcium	14 mg	Iron	2.43 mg
Magnesium	32 mg	Phosphorus	113 mg
Potassium	356 mg	Zinc	1.1 mg
Thiamine	0.066 mg	Riboflavin	0.02 mg
Niacin	0.54 mg	Pantothenic acid	1.014 mg
Vitamin B_6	0.05 mg	Vitamin C	3.3 mg

- High in saturated fats essential for better health.
- Saturated fatty acid in the coconut is lauric acid which increases HDL cholesterol levels in the blood.
- Coconut water is refreshing drink in summer thirst. It contains simple sugar, electrolytes, minerals and bioactive compounds.
- Very good source of folic acid, riboflavin, niacin, thiamin and pyridoxine.
- Contains good amount of potassium.
- Coconut oil is an excellent emollient agent.
- Coconut water is an anti-ageing, anti-carcinogenic, and anti-thrombotic.
- Excellent source of copper, calcium, iron, manganese, magnesium and zinc.

LEMON

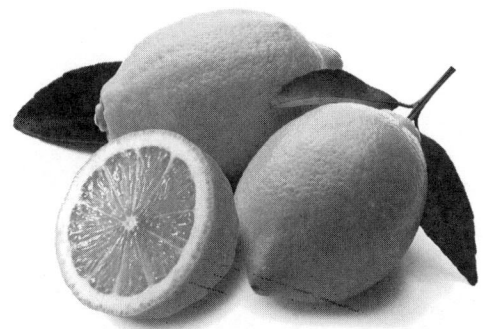

(Per 100 gm)			
Energy	29 kcal	Carbohydrates	9.32 g
Sugars	2.5 g	Dietary fiber	2.8 g
Fat	0.3 g	Protein	1.1 g
Calcium	26 mg	Iron	0.6 mg
Magnesium	8 mg	Manganese	0.03 mg
Phosphorus	16 mg	Potassium	138 mg
Zinc	0.06 mg	Thiamine	0.04 mg
Riboflavin	0.02 mg	Niacin	0.1 mg
Pantothenic acid	0.19 mg	Vitamin B_6	0.08 mg
Folic acid	11 μg	Choline	5.1 mg
Vitamin C	53 mg		

- With hot water is effective digestive disorders, nausea, heartburn and biliousness.
- Useful in constipation and worm infestations.
- Regular consumption of lemon juice in the morning stimulates the bile-producing capacity of liver.
- Juice is helpful in dissolving gall bladder stones.
- Coffee and lemon juice mixture useful in treatment of malaria and headaches.
- Lemon juice applied to nostrils controls epistaxis.
- Also stops gum bleeding if applied locally.
- Useful in treatment of asthma, tonsillitis and sore throat.
- Fastens healing of wounds

- Drops of lemon juice in bath water increases freshness.
- It is diuretic and useful in treatment of urinary tract infections.
- In treatment of arthritis and chapped lips.

ARECA NUT (Betel Nut)

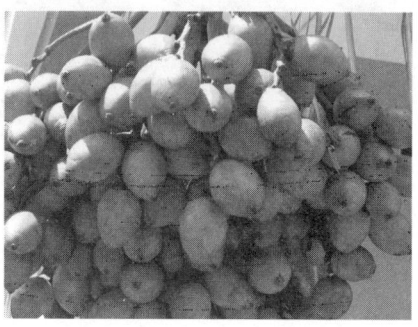

APRICOT

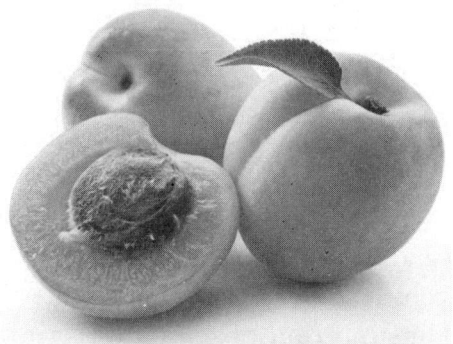

- Golden eggs of the sun.
- Low in calories.
- Rich source of dietary fiber, antioxidants, vitamins and minerals.
- Prevent heart disease by reducing LDL.
- Protection against malignancies.
- Excellent sources of vitamin A and carotenes.
- Rich in vitamin C

(Per 100 gm)			
Energy	50 kcal	Carbohydrates	11 g
Protein	1.4 g	Fat	0.4 g
Cholesterol	0 mg	Fiber	2 g
Sodium	1 mg	Potassium	259 mg
Calcium	13 mg	Iron	0.39 mg
Magnesium	10 mg	Manganese	0.077 mg
Phosphorus	23 mg	Zinc	0.2 mg
Folic acid	9 µg	Niacin	0.600 mg
Pantothenic acid	0.240 mg	Pyridoxine	0.054 mg
Riboflavin	0.040 mg	Thiamin	0.030 mg
Vitamin A	1926 IU	Vitamin C	10 mg
Vitamin E	0 mg	Vitamin K	3.3 µg
Lutein-zeaxanthin	89 µg		

- Good source of potassium, iron, zinc, calcium and manganese
- Rich in zeaxanthin that protect eyes from age-related macular disease.

CHERIMOYA FRUIT

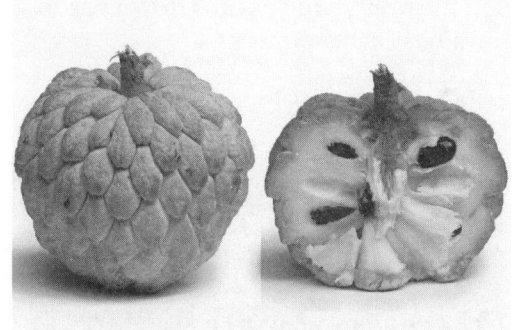

- Have very sweet and pleasant flavor.
- No saturated fats or cholesterol.
- Good amount of dietary fiber
- Prevent absorption of cholesterol in the gut.
- Fiber protects the mucous membrane from malignancy-causing chemicals in the colon.

(Per 100 gm)			
Energy	75 kcal	Carbohydrates	17.71 g
Protein	1.57 g	Fat	0.68 g
Cholesterol	0 mg	Dietary fiber	3 g
Sodium	7 mg	Potassium	287 mg
Calcium	10 mg	Copper	0.069 mg
Iron	0.27 mg	Magnesium	17 mg
Manganese	0.093 mg	Phosphorus	26 mg
Zinc	0.16 mg	Folic acid	23 µg
Niacin	0.644 mg	Pantothenic acid	0.345 mg
Pyridoxine	0.257 mg	Riboflavin	0.131 mg
Thiamin	0.101 mg	Vitamin A	5 IU
Vitamin C	12.6 mg	Vitamin E	0.27 mg

- Have anti-malignancy, anti-malarial, and anti-helminthes properties.
- Very good in vitamin C which gives resistance against infectious agents and harmful pro-inflammatory free radicals.
- In this fruit there is well balanced sodium–potassium ratio.
- Rich in copper, magnesium, iron and manganese.
- Good source of vitamin B_6 that keep-up GABA neuro chemical in the brain which calms down nervous irritability, tension, and headache ailments.

CHOKEBERRY (Aronia)

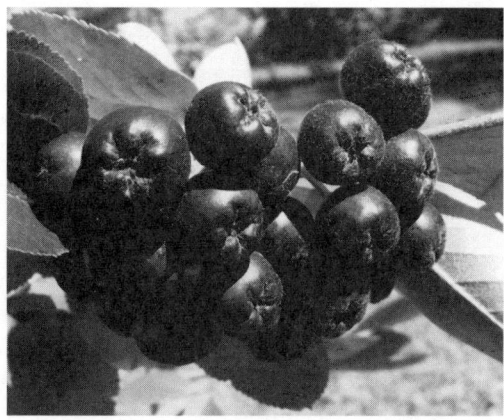

(Per 100 gm)			
Energy	47 kcal	Carbohydrates	9.6 g
Protein	1.4 g	Fat	0.5 g
Cholesterol	0 mg	Dietary fiber	5.3 g
Folic acid	25 µg	Vitamin A	214 IU
Vitamin C	21 mg	Vitamin E	1.17 mg
Vitamin K	19.8 µg	Sodium	1 mg
Potassium	162 mg	Calcium	30 mg
Iron	0.62 mg	Magnesium	20 mg
Manganese	0.646 mg	Zinc	0.53 mg
Phyto-nutrients			
Carotene-α	0 µg	Carotene-β	128 µg
Lutein-zeaxanthin	118 µg		

- Low in calories and fats.
- Contains high quantity of phenolic flavonoid phyto-chemical-anthocyanins which decreases risk against malignancy, aging and neurological diseases, inflammation, diabetes and bacterial infections.
- Rich in flavonoid antioxidants such as carotenes, luteins and zeaxanthins which protects eyes from age-related macular disease.
- Good source of antioxidants like vitamins C, A, E, beta-carotene, folic acid, potassium, iron and manganese.

CRANBERRIES

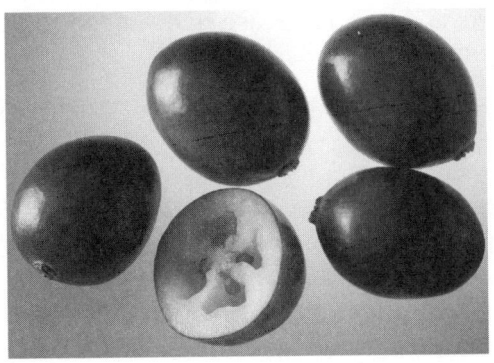

(Per 100 gm)			
Energy	46 kcal	Carbohydrates	12.2 g
Protein	0.4 g	Fat	0.13 g
Cholesterol	0 mg	Dietary fiber	4.6 g
Sodium	2 mg	Potassium	85 mg
Calcium	8 mg	Copper	0.061 mg
Iron	0.25 mg	Magnesium	6 mg
Manganese	0.360 mg	Phosphorus	13 mg
Selenium	0.1 µg	Zinc	0.10 mg
Folic acid	1 µg	Niacin	0.101 mg
Pantothenic acid	0.295 mg	Pyridoxine	0.057 mg
Riboflavin	0.020 mg	Thiamin	0.012 mg
Vitamin A	60 IU	Vitamin C	13.3 mg
Vitamin E	1.20 mg	Vitamin K	5.1 µg

- High amount of phenolic flavonoid phytochemicals–pro-anthocyanidins which has benefits against malignancy, neurological diseases, inflammation, diabetes and bacterial infections.
- Gives protection against gram-negative bacterial infections.
- Prevents plaque and cavity formation on the tooth.
- Prevents urinary tract infection.
- Rich in vitamins C, A, β-carotene, lutein, zeaxanthin, folic acid, potassium and manganese.
- Contains antioxidant like oligomeric proanthocyanidins, anthocyanidin flavonoids, cyanidin, peonidin and quercetin which prevents cardiovascular diseases by lowering LDL cholesterol levels and increase HDL—good cholesterol levels in the blood.

DURIAN FRUIT

- Rich in energy, minerals and vitamins.
- Easily digestible flesh contains simple sugars like fructose and sucrose that when eaten replenish energy and revitalize the body instantly.
- Contains high amount of fats—free from saturated fats and cholesterol.

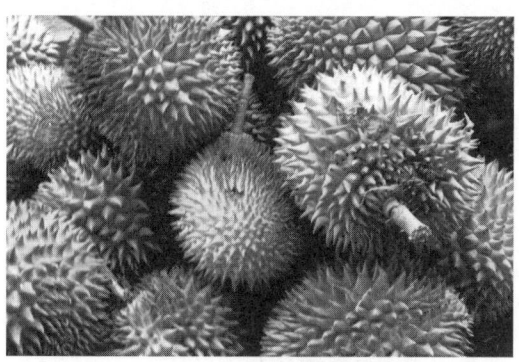

(Per 100 gm)			
Energy	147 kcal	Carbohydrates	27.09 g
Protein	1.47 g	Fat	5.33 g
Cholesterol	0 mg	Dietary fiber	3.8 g
Folic acid	36 mcg	Sodium	2 mg
Potassium	436 mg	Calcium	6 mg
Copper	0.207 mg	Iron	0.43 mg
Magnesium	30 mg	Manganese	0.325 mg
Phosphorus	39 mg	Zinc	0.28 mg
Niacin	1.074 mg	Pantothenic acid	0.230 mg
Pyridoxine	0.316 mg	Riboflavin	0.200 mg
Thiamin	0.374 mg	Vitamin A	44 IU
Vitamin C	19.7 mg		

- High levels of essential amino acid, tryptophan—these neuro-chemicals have important function in sleep induction and in treatment of epilepsy.
- Rich source of potassium which controls heart rate and blood pressure.
- Rich in dietary fiber which helps to protect the colon by malignancy-causing chemicals.
- A good source of antioxidant like vitamin C which helps the body develop resistance against infectious agents and harmful free radicals.
- Rich in niacin, riboflavin, pantothenic acid , pyridoxine and thiamin.
- Rich in manganese, copper, iron and magnesium.

GOOSEBERRIES—AAMLA

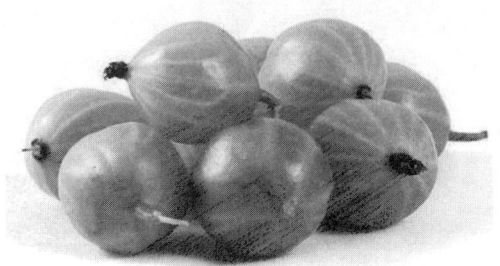

(Per 100 gm)			
Energy	44 kcal	Carbohydrates	10.18 g
Protein	0.88 g	Fat	0.58 g
Dietary fiber	4.3 g	Sodium	1 mg
Potassium	198 mg	Calcium	25 mg
Copper	0.070 mg	Iron	0.31 mg
Magnesium	10 mg	Manganese	0.144 mg
Phosphorus	27 mg	Folic acid	6 mcg
Niacin	0.300 mg	Pantothenic acid	0.286 mg
Pyridoxine	0.080 mg	Riboflavin	0.030 mg
Thiamin	0.040 mg	Vitamin A	290 IU
Vitamin C	27.7 mg		

- Low in calories.
- High amount of phenolic phytochemicals—flavones and anthocyanins which have effects against malignancy, aging, inflammation and neurological diseases.
- Protects from lung and oral cavity malignancies.
- Small amount of pyridoxine, pantothenic acid, folic acid and thiamin.
- Rich source of copper, calcium, phosphorus, manganese, magnesium and potassium.
- Moderate source of vitamin C which gives immunity against infections and harmful oxygen free radicals.
- Small amount of vitamin A which maintains the integrity of mucus membranes and skin.

JACKFRUIT

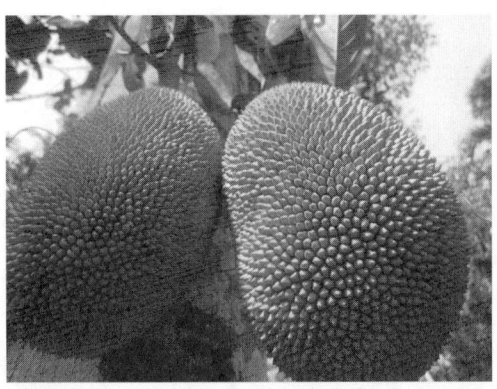

(Per 100 gm)			
Energy	95 kcal	Carbohydrates	23.5 g
Protein	1.72 g	Fat	0.64 g
Cholesterol	0 mg	Dietary fiber	1.5 g
Sodium	3 mg	Potassium	303 mg
Calcium	34 mg	Iron	0.60 mg
Magnesium	37 mg	Manganese	0.197 mg
Phosphorus	36 mg	Phosphorus	21 mg
Selenium	0.6 mg	Zinc	0.42 mg
Folic acid	24 µg	Niacin	0.920 mg
Pyridoxine	0.329 mg	Riboflavin	0.055 mg
Thiamin	0.105 mg	Vitamin A	110 IU
Vitamin C	13.7 mg	Vitamin E	0.34 mg

- Soft, easily digestible flesh contains simple sugars like fructose and sucrose that replenishes energy and revitalizes the body instantly.
- Rich in dietary fiber which is useful as bulk laxative in constipation and also protects the colon mucous membrane from malignancy-causing chemicals.
- Good amounts of vitamin B_6, niacin, riboflavin and folic acid.
- Good source of potassium, magnesium, manganese and iron.
- Contains small amount of vitaminA, and flavonoid pigments such as carotene-β, xanthin, lutein and cryptoxanthin-β. These

are useful as antioxidants and visual functions. Also protects from lung and oral cavity malignancies.

• Good source of antioxidant like vitamin C which gives resistance against infections and harmful free radicals.

JACKFRUIT SEEDS

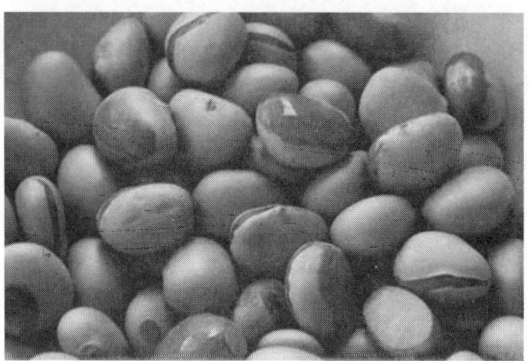

Rich in protein and nutritious.

KUMQUAT FRUIT

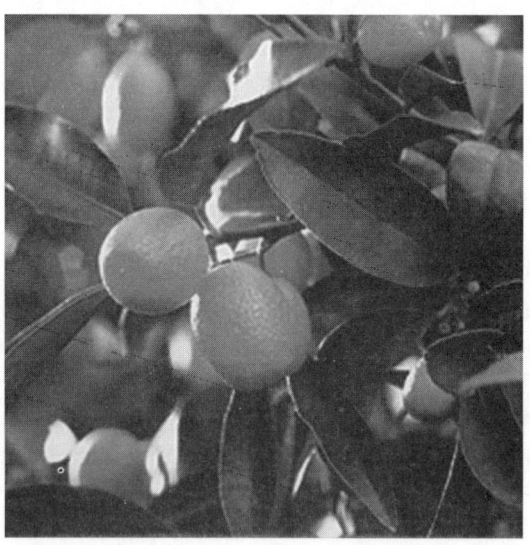

(Per 100 gm)			
Energy	71 kcal	Carbohydrates	15.90 g
Protein	1.88 g	Fat	0.86 g
Cholesterol	0 mg	Dietary fiber	6.5 g
Sodium	10 mg	Potassium	186 mg
Calcium	62 mg	Copper	0.095 mg
Iron	0.86 mg	Magnesium	20 mg
Manganese	0.135 mg	Selenium	0.0 mcg
Zinc	0.17 mg	Folic acid	17 µg
Niacin	0.429 mg	Pantothenic acid	0.208 mg
Pyridoxine	0.036 mg	Riboflavin	0.090 mg
Thiamin	0.037 mg	Vitamin A	290 IU
Vitamin C	43.9 mg	Vitamin E	0.15 mg
Vitamin K	0 µg		

- Rich in many essential oils, antioxidants and fiber.
- Contains poly-phenolic flavonoid antioxidants such as carotenes, lutein, zeaxanthin and tannins.
- Rich in vitamins A, C and E which give protection from malignancies, diabetes, degenerative diseases and infections.
- Rich in vitamin C which has role in prevention of neuro-degenerative diseases, arthritis and diabetes.
- Rich source of thiamin, niacin, pyridoxine, folic acid and pantothenic acid.
- Rich source of calcium, copper, potassium, manganese, iron, selenium and zinc.

LOQUAT FRUIT

- Low in calories.
- Rich in insoluble dietary fiber—pectin which protects the colon mucous membrane from malignancy-causing chemicals and also reduces blood cholesterol levels.
- Excellent source of vitamin A which maintains integrity of mucus membranes and skin, also gives protection from lung and oral cavity malignancies.
- Very rich source of potassium and folic acid, vitamin B_6 and niacin and small amount of vitamin C.
- Good source of iron, copper and calcium, manganese.

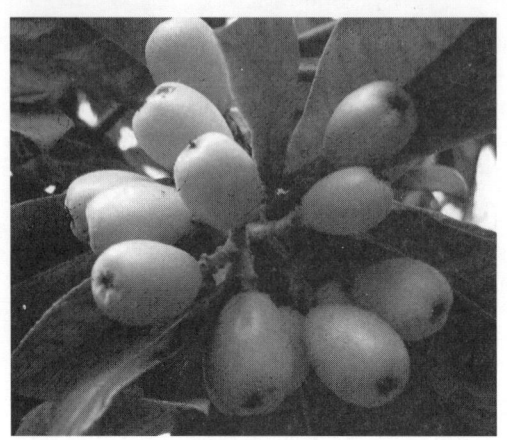

(Per 100 gm)			
Energy	47 kcal	Carbohydrates	12.14 g
Protein	0.43 g	Fat	0.20 g
Dietary fiber	1.70 g	Folic acid	14 µg
Niacin	0.180 mg	Pyridoxine	0.100 mg
Riboflavin	0.024 mg	Thiamin	0.019 mg
Vitamin A	1528 IU	Vitamin C	1 mg
Sodium	1 mg	Potassium	266 mg
Calcium	16 mg	Copper	0.040 mg
Iron	0.28 mg	Magnesium	13 mg
Manganese	0.148 mg	Phosphorus	27 mg
Selenium	0.6 µg	Zinc	0.05 mg

MANGOSTEEN

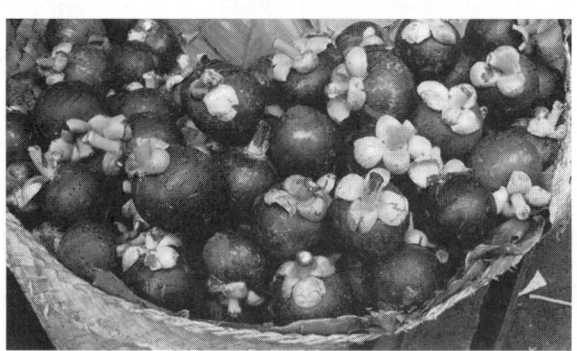

- Very delicious and juicy
- Low in calories
- Very good amount of copper, manganese and magnesium which gives protection against stroke and coronary heart diseases.
- Good source of vitamin C which is powerful water soluble antioxidant.
- Moderate source of thiamin, niacin and folic acid.

(Per 100 gm)			
Energy	63 kcal	Carbohydrates	15.6 g
Protein	0.50 g	Fat	0.4 g
Cholesterol	0 mg	Dietary fiber	5.10 g
Sodium	7 mg	Potassium	48 mg
Calcium	5.49 mg	Copper	0.069 mg
Iron	0.17 mg	Magnesium	13.9 mg
Manganese	0.10 mg	Phosphorus	9.21 mg
Zinc	0.12 mg	Folic acid	31 µg
Niacin	0.286 mg	Pantothenic acid	0.032 mg
Pyridoxine	0.041 mg	Riboflavin	0.054 mg
Thiamin	0.054 mg	Vitamin A	35 IU
Vitamin C	7.2 mg		

MULBERRIES

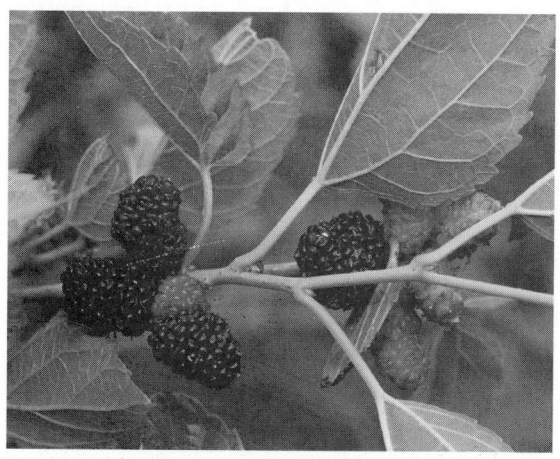

(Per 100 gm)			
Energy	43 kcal	Carbohydrates	9.80 g
Protein	1.44 g	Fat	0.39 g
Cholesterol	0 mg	Dietary fiber	1.7 g
Sodium	10 mg	Potassium	194 mg
Calcium	39 mg	Copper	60 µg
Iron	1.85 mg	Magnesium	18 mg
Selenium	0.6 µg	Zinc	0.12 mg
Folic acid	6 µg	Niacin	0.620 mg
Pyridoxine	0.050 mg	Riboflavin	0.101 mg
Vitamin A	25 IU	Vitamin C	36.4 mg
Vitamin E	0.87 mg	Vitamin K	7.8 µg

- Low in calories.
- Good source of potassium, manganese, and magnesium.
- Rich in B-complex group of vitamins and vitamin K.
- Contains resveratrol which gives protection against stroke.
- Excellent source of vitamin C which gives protection against infection, inflammation and harmful free radicals.
- Small amount of vitamins A and E .
- Contains dietary carotenoid zeaxanthin which selectively concentrates into the retinal macula lutea and gives protection to the retina from the harmful ultraviolet rays.
- High quantity of phenolics flavonoids phytochemicals—anthocyanins which has effects against malignancy, neurological diseases, inflammation, diabetes and bacterial infections.
- Excellent source of iron.

OLIVES

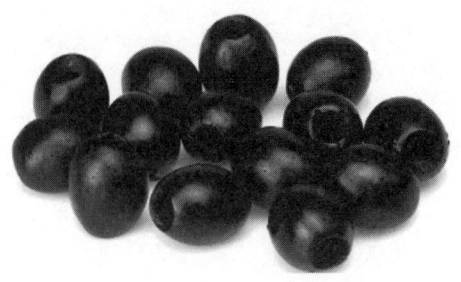

(Per 100 gm)			
Energy	115 kcal	Carbohydrates	6.26 g
Protein	0.84 g	Fat	10.68 g
Cholesterol	0 mg	Dietary fiber	3.2 g
Sodium	735 mg	Potassium	8 mg
Calcium	88 mg	Copper	0.251 mg
Iron	3.30 mg	Magnesium	4 mg
Manganese	0.020 mg	Phosphorus	3 mg
Selenium	0.9 µg	Zinc	0.22 mg
Folic acid	0 µg	Niacin	0.037 mg
Pantothenic acid	0.015 mg	Pyridoxine	0.009 mg
Riboflavin	0 mg	Thiamin	0.003 mg
Vitamin A	403 IU	Vitamin C	0.9
Vitamin E	1.65 mg	Vitamin K	1.4 µg

- Moderate source of calorie.
- Fat is of mono-unsaturated fatty acids like oleic acid and palmitoleic acid that helps to lower LDL or "bad cholesterol" and increase HDL or "good cholesterol" which prevents coronary artery disease and strokes.
- Rich in calcium, copper, iron, manganese, zinc, niacin, choline, and pantothenic acid.
- Healthiest edible oils having less saturated fat and composes linoleic (omega-6) and linolenic acids (omega-3) as essential fatty acids.
- It contains tyrosol phenolic compounds—oleuropein and oleocanthal which gives protection against malignancy, inflammation, coronary artery disease, degenerative nerve diseases and diabetes.
- Contains good amount of vitamin E which maintains the integrity of cell membrane of mucus membranes and skin by harmful oxygen-free radicals

PASSION FRUIT

- Delicious fruit
- Rich source of antioxidants, minerals, vitamins and fiber.
- Good source of dietary fiber which removes cholesterol from the body.

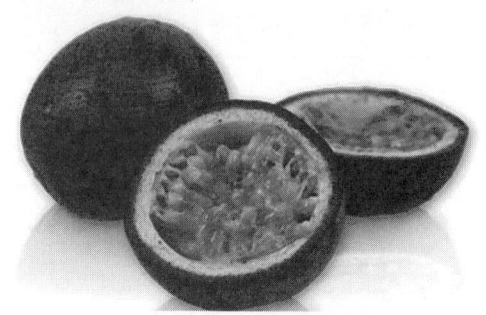

(Per 100 gm)			
Energy	97 kcal	Carbohydrates	23.38 g
Protein	2.20 g	Fat	0.70 g
Cholesterol	0 mg	Dietary fiber	10.40 g
Sodium	0 mg	Potassium	348 mg
Calcium	12 mg	Copper	0.086 mg
Iron	1.60 mg	Magnesium	29 mg
Phosphorus	68 mg	Selenium	0.6 µg
Zinc	0.10 µg	Folic acid	14 µg
Niacin	1.500 mg	Pyridoxine	0.100 mg
Riboflavin	0.130 mg	Thiamin	0.00 mg
Vitamin A	1274 IU	Vitamin C	30 mg
Vitamin E	0.02 µg	Vitamin K	0.7 mg

- Good levels of vitamin A and flavonoid antioxidants such as β-carotene and cryptoxanthin-β which is good for healthy eyesight.
- Protects lung and oral cavity from malignancies.
- Rich in potassium, which regulates heart rate and blood pressure.
- Good source of iron, copper, magnesium and phosphorus.
- Rich source of dietary insoluble fiber which acts as a bulk laxative in constipation and protects the colon mucous membrane from malignancy-causing chemicals.
- Good in vitamin C which gives resistance against flu-like infectious agents and pro-inflammatory free radicals.

PEACHES

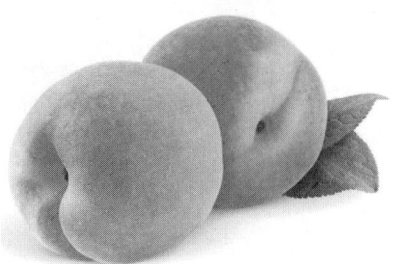

(Per 100 gm)			
Energy	39 kcal	Carbohydrates	9.54 g
Protein	0.91 g	Fat	0.25 g
Cholesterol	0 mg	Dietary fiber	1.5 g
Sodium	0 mg	Potassium	190 mg
Calcium	6 mg	Copper	0.068 mg
Iron	0.25 mg	Magnesium	9 mg
Manganese	0.61 mg	Phosphorus	11 mg
Zinc	0.17 mg	Folic acid	4 µg
Niacin	0.806 mg	Pantothenic acid	0.153 mg
Pyridoxine	0.025 mg	Riboflavin	0.031 mg
Thiamin	0.024 mg	Vitamin A	326 IU
Vitamin C	6.6 mg	Vitamin E	0.73 mg
Vitamin K	2.6 µg		

- Low in calories and contain no saturated fats.
- Rich in potassium, fluoride and iron.
- Contains health promoting flavonoid polyphenolic anti-oxidants such as lutein, zeaxanthin and β-cryptoxanthin which has role in aging and various disease processes.
- Moderate source of vitamin C—antioxidant which gives protection against infectious agents and harmful free radicals.
- Moderate source of vitamin A and β-carotene which gives protection from lung and oral cavity malignancies.

PEARS

- Good source of dietary fiber which gives protection against colon malignancy, also act as bulk laxative.

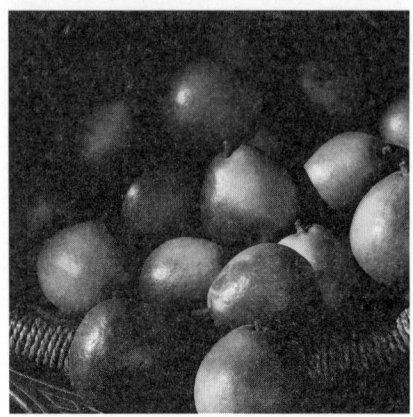

(Per 100 gm)			
Energy	58 kcal	Carbohydrates	13.81 g
Protein	0.38 g	Fat	0.12 g
Cholesterol	0 mg	Dietary fiber	3.10 g
Vitamins		Folic acid	7 µg
Niacin	0.157 mg	Pantothenic acid	0.048 mg
Pyridoxine	0.028 mg	Riboflavin	0.025 mg
Thiamin	0.012 mg	Vitamin A	23 IU
Vitamin C	4.2 mg	Vitamin E	0.12 mg
Vitamin K	4.5 µg	Sodium	1 mg
Potassium	119 mg	Calcium	9 mg
Copper	0.082 mg	Iron	0.17 mg
Magnesium	7 mg	Phosphorus	11 mg
Zinc	0.10 mg		

- Very low calorie fruits so useful for reduction in weight.
- Decreases blood LDL cholesterol.
- Good quantities of vitamin C.
- Good sources of antioxidant flavonoids phyto-nutrients such as beta-carotene, lutein and zeaxanthin.
- Good source of copper, iron, potassium, manganese, magnesium, folic acid, riboflavin and pyridoxine.
- Useful in treating colitis, chronic gallbladder disorders, arthritis and gout.

TANGERINES

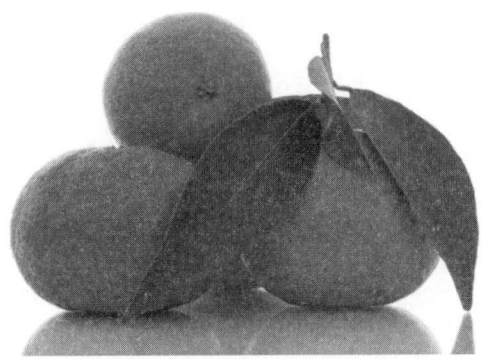

(Per 100 gm)			
Energy	53 kcal	Carbohydrates	13.34 g
Protein	0.81 g	Fat	0.31 g
Cholesterol	0 mg	Dietary fiber	1.8 g
Folic acid	16 µg	Niacin	0.376 mg
Pantothenic acid	0.216 mg	Pyridoxine	0.078 mg
Riboflavin	0.036 mg	Thiamin	0.058 mg
Vitamin C	26.7 mg	Vitamin A	681 IU
Vitamin E	0.20 mg	Vitamin K	0 µg
Sodium	2 mg	Potassium	166 mg
Calcium	37 mg	Copper	42 µg
Iron	0.15 mg	Magnesium	12 mg
Manganese	0.039 mg	Zinc	0.07 mg

- Very low in calories.
- Rich sources of vitamin C—a natural antioxidant which prevents from neurodegenerative diseases and arthritis.
- Contains phyto-chemical antioxidants which protects from malignancies, arthritis, obesity and coronary heart diseases.
- Contains natural soluble and insoluble fiber hemi-cellulose and pectin which prevents cholesterol absorption in the gut and also acts as a laxative.
- Rich in vitamins and minerals.

RASPBERRY

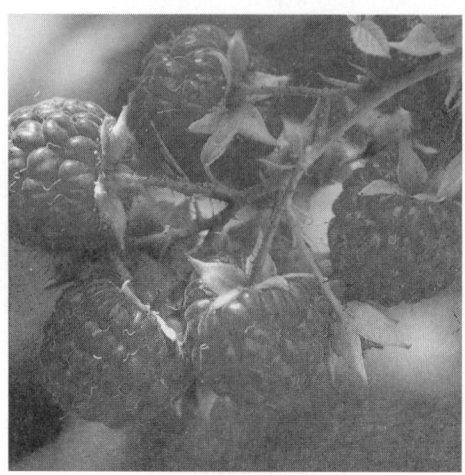

(Per 100 gm)			
Energy	52 kcal	Carbohydrates	11.94 g
Protein	1.20 g	Fat	0.65 g
Cholesterol	0 mg	Dietary fiber	6.5 g
Folic acid	21 mcg	Niacin	0.598 mg
Pyridoxine	0.055 mg	Riboflavin	0.038 mg
Vitamin A	33 IU	Vitamin C	26.2 mg
Vitamin E	1.42 mg	Vitamin K	7.8 g
Sodium	1 mg	Potassium	151 mg
Calcium	25 mg	Copper	90 g
Iron	0.69 mg	Magnesium	22 mg
Manganese	0.670 mg	Zinc	0.42 mg

- Low in calories and saturated fats.
- Rich source of dietary fiber and antioxidants.
- High levels of phenolic flavonoid phytochemicals such as anthocyanins, ellagic acid quercetin, gallic acid, cyanidins, pelargonidins, catechins, kaempferol and salicylic acid which gives protection against malignancy, aging, inflammation and neuro-degenerative diseases.
- It contains a low-calorie sugar—xylitol which is helpful in diabetics.

- Excellent source of vitamin C—a powerful natural antioxidant useful against inflammation and harmful free radicals.
- Rich in vitamins A and E.
- Good amount of potassium, manganese, copper, iron and magnesium.
- Very good amount of vitamin B_6, niacin, riboflavin and folic acid.

QUINCE FRUIT

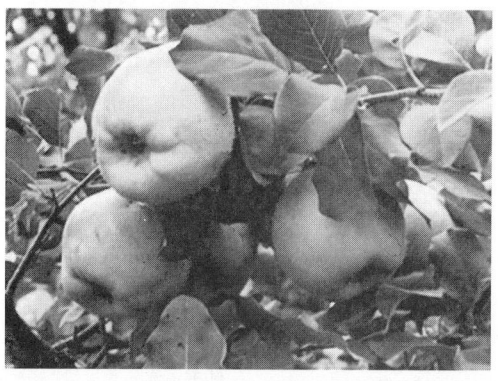

(Per 100 gm)			
Energy	57 kcal	Carbohydrates	13.81 g
Protein	0.40 g	Fat	0.10 g
Cholesterol	0 mg	Dietary fiber	1.9 g
Sodium	1 mg	Potassium	119 mg
Calcium	11 mg	Copper	0.130 mg
Iron	0.70 mg	Magnesium	8 mg
Phosphorus	11 mg	Selenium	0.6 µg
Zinc	0.04 mg	Folic acid	3 µg
Niacin	0.200 mg	Pantothenic acid	0.081 mg
Pyridoxine	0.040 mg	Riboflavin	0.030 mg
Thiamin	0.020 mg	Vitamin A	40 IU
Vitamin C	15 mg	Vitamin E	0.12 mg
Vitamin K	4.5 µg		

- Low calorie fruit.
- Pulp along with its peel contains good amount of fiber that helps to reduce body weight and blood LDL cholesterol levels.
- It contains caffeoylquinic acid, procyanidin B_2, oligomeric procyanidin, polymeric procyanidin and essential oils like furfural, limonene, linalol, vomifoliol, toluene, β-ionone, α-terpineol. These have typical unique fragrance.
- Good concentration of vitamin C which boosts up immunity, reduces viral episodes and inflammatory conditions.
- Good source of copper, iron, potassium and magnesium, thiamin, riboflavin and pyridoxine.
- Anti-allergenic and anti-inflammatory properties.
- Useful in treatment of cystitis and atopic dermatitis.

PLUMS

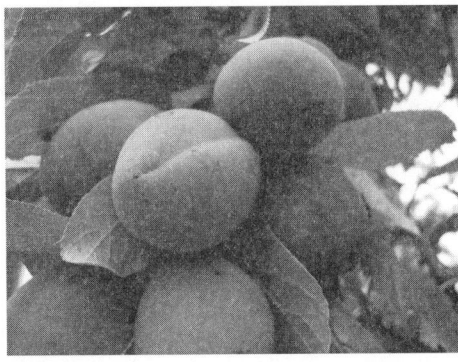

- Delicious, fleshy fruit.
- Low in calories.
- No saturated fats.
- Rich in dietary fiber, sorbitol, and satin relieves constipation.
- Rich in potassium, fluoride, iron, niacin, vitamin B_6, pantothenic acid, vitamin K which reduces risk of Alzheimer's disease.
- Moderate source of vitamin C—a powerful natural antioxidant.

(Per 100 gm)			
Energy	46 kcal	Carbohydrates	11.42 g
Protein	0.70 g	Fat	0.28 g
Cholesterol	0 mg	Dietary fiber	1.40 g
Sodium	1 mg	Potassium	157 mg
Calcium	6 mg	Copper	0.057 mg
Iron	0.17 mg	Magnesium	7 mg
Manganese	0.052 mg	Phosphorus	16 mg
Selenium	1.0 µg	Zinc	0.10 mg
Folic acid	5 µg	Niacin	0.417 mg
Pantothenic acid	0.135 mg	Pyridoxine	0.029 mg
Riboflavin	0.026 mg	Thiamin	0.028 mg
Vitamin A	345 IU	Vitamin C	9.5 mg
Vitamin E	0.26 mg	Vitamin K	6.4 µg

- Moderate source of vitamin A and beta carotene—essential for good eyesight.

SAPODILLA (Sapota)

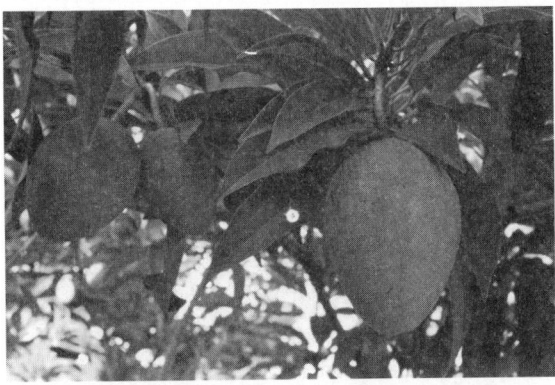

- Rich calories.
- Good source of dietary fiber which acts as bulk laxative useful in constipation and also protects mucous membrane of the colon from malignancy-causing toxins.
- Good source of potassium, copper, iron, folic acid, niacin and pantothenic acid.

(Per 100 gm)			
Energy	83 kcal	Carbohydrates	19.9 g
Protein	0.44 g	Fat	1.10 g
Cholesterol	0 mg	Dietary fiber	5.3 g
Sodium	12 mg	Potassium	193 mg
Calcium	21 mg	Copper	0.086 mg
Iron	0.80 mg	Magnesium	12 mg
Phosphorous	12 mg	Selenium	0.6 µg
Zinc	0.10 mg	Folic acid	14 µg
Niacin	0.200 mg	Pantothenic acid	0.252 mg
Pyridoxine	0.037 mg	Riboflavin	0.020 mg
Thiamin	0.058 mg	Vitamin A	60 IU
Vitamin C	14.7 mg		

- Rich in antioxidant polyphenolic compound tannin which has anti-inflammatory, antiviral, anti-bacterial and anti-parasitic effects.
- Good amount of vitamins C and A.

PERSIMMON FRUIT

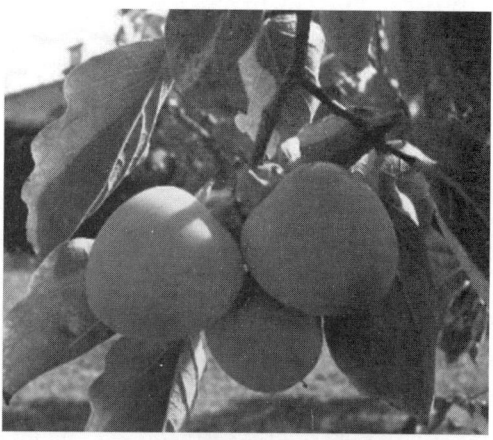

- Low in calories and fats.
- Contains phyto-nutrients, flavonoid polyphenolic anti-oxidants like catechins and gallocatechins.
- Very good source of vitamin C, powerful antioxidant.

(Per 100 gm)			
Energy	70 kcal	Carbohydrates	18.59 g
Protein	0.58 g	Fat	0.19 g
Cholesterol	0 g	Dietary fiber	3.6 g
Choline	7.6 mg	Sodium	1 mg
Potassium	161 mg	Calcium	8 mg
Copper	0.113 mg	Iron	0.15 mg
Magnesium	9 mg	Manganese	0.355 mg
Phosphorus	17 mg	Zinc	0.11 mg
Folic acid	8 µg	Niacin	0.100 mg
Pyridoxine	0.100 mg	Riboflavin	0.020 mg
Thiamin	0.030 mg	Vitamin C	7.5 mg
Vitamin A	81 IU	Vitamin E	0.73 mg
Vitamin K	2.6 µg		

- Rich folic acid, pyridoxine and thiamin.
- Rich potassium, manganese, copper and phosphorus.
- Contains antioxidants like vitamin A, beta-carotene, lycopene, lutein, zeaxanthin and cryptoxanthin.
- Contains zeaxanthin a dietary carotenoid, which is selectively absorbed into the retinal macula lutea in the eyes gives protection against age-related macular disease.

LIMONIA ACIDISSIMA (Wood Apple)

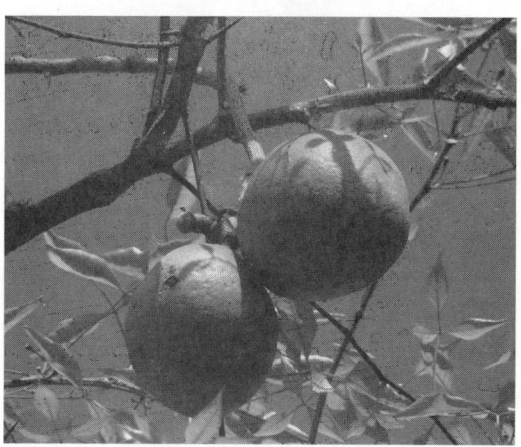

(Per 100 gm)			
Energy	140 calories	Carbohydrate	31 gm
Protein	2 gm		
Rich in beta-carotene			
Rich in thiamine, riboflavin and vitamin C			
Rich in oxalic, malic, citric acid and tannic acid			

- Good for digestion. It destroys intestinal worms and cures chronic dysentery.
- Prevents post-partum depression.
- With honey prevents breast and uterine malignancy.
- Cures sterility.
- Useful in treatment of piles or stomach ulcers, diarrhea and indigestion.
- Cures scurvy.
- Gum on tree is helpful in treatment of diabetes, leaves can cure sore throat, chronic cough.
- A wood apple chutney made with salt and tamarind can cure hiccups.

CUSTARD APPLE

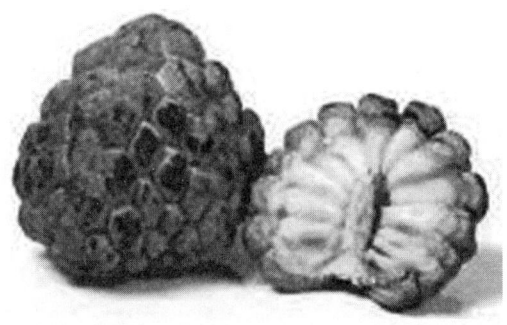

(Per 100 gm)			
Energy	101 Calories	Fat	0.6 gm
Sodium	4 mg	Carbohydrates	25.2 gm
Dietary fiber	2.4 gm	Sugars	0.0 gm
Protein	1.7 gm		

- Rich in vitamin C—an antioxidant which helps in neutralizing free radicals.
- Rich in potassium and vitamin B_6.
- Also contains copper
- Rich in vitamin A—good for hair, eyes and healthy skin.
- Rich in magnesium, which has role in relaxing muscles and protecting heart.
- Rich source of dietary fiber, which helps in digestion.
- For treating diarrhea and dysentery.
- Acts as expectorant, stimulant, coolant and haematinic.
- Seeds are insecticidal and abortifacient.

ANNONA SQUAMOSA (Sugar-Apple)

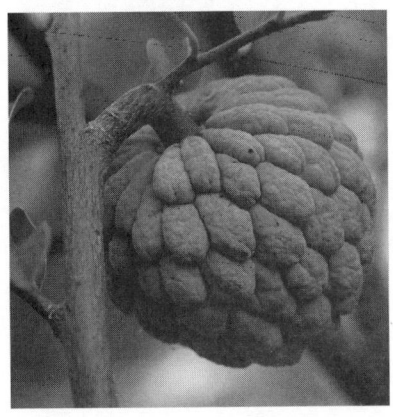

(Per 100 gm)			
Energy	94 kcal	Carbohydrates	23.64 g
Dietary fiber	4.4 g	Fat	0.29 g
Protein	2.06 g	Calcium	24 mg
Iron	0.6 mg	Magnesium	21 mg
Manganese	0.42 mg	Phosphorus	32 mg
Potassium	247 mg	Sodium	9 mg
Zinc	0.1 mg	Thiamine	0.11 mg
Riboflavin	0.113 mg	Niacin	0.883 mg
Pantothenic acid	0.226 mg	Vitamin B_6	0.2 mg
Folic acid	14 µg	Vitamin C	36.3 mg

- Contains good amount of vitamin C—strengthen the immune system and fights malignancy-causing free radicals.
- Rich in phosphorus—formation of bones and teeth
- Contains carnitine which decreases bad cholesterol levels.
- Rich in lysine which is useful in skin tightening and facial wrinkling.

GOOSEBERRIES

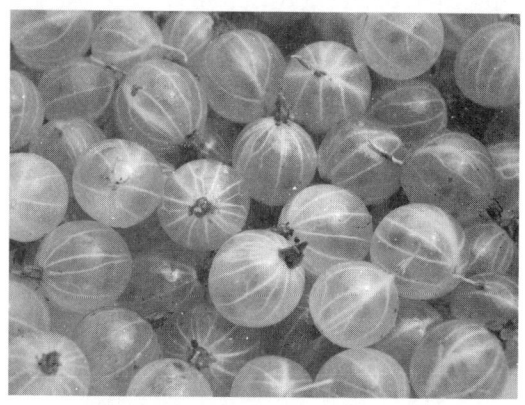

(Per 150 gm)			
Energy	66 calories	Fat	0.9 g
Sodium	2 mg	Carbohydrates	15.3 g
Dietary fiber	6.5 g	Protein	1.3 g

ALMOND

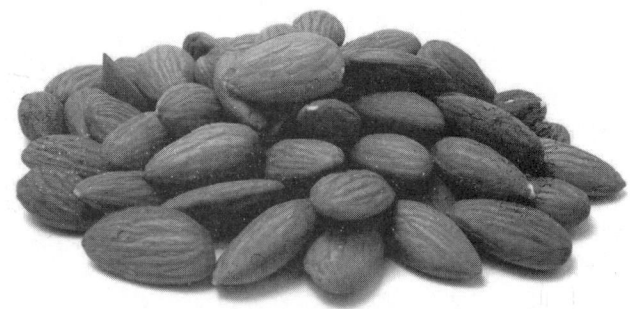

(Per 100 gm)			
Energy	575 kcal	Carbohydrates	21.67 g
Protein	21.22 g	Fat	49.42 g
Cholesterol	0 mg	Dietary fiber	12.20 g
Sodium	1 mg	Potassium	705 mg
Calcium	264 mg	Copper	0.996 mg
Iron	3.72 mg	Magnesium	268 mg
Manganese	2.285 mg	Phosphorus	484 mg
Selenium	2.5 µg	Zinc	3.08 mg
Folic acid	50 µg	Niacin	3.385 mg
Pantothenic acid	0.47 mg	Pyridoxine	0.143 mg
Riboflavin	1.014 mg	Thiamin	0.211 mg
Vitamin A	1 IU	Vitamin C	0 mg
Vitamin E	26 mg		

- Rich in dietary fiber, vitamins, and minerals
- Complete source of energy.
- Rich in mono-unsaturated fatty acids like oleic and palmitoleic acids which helps to lower LDL or "bad cholesterol" and increase HDL or "good cholesterol."
- Rich in manganese, potassium, calcium, iron, magnesium, zinc and selenium.
- Almond oil is as an emollient which keeps skin moist.
- Medicines in aromatherapy, in pharmaceutical, and cosmetic industries.
- Excellent source of vitamin E—a powerful lipid soluble antioxidant, required for maintaining cell membrane integrity.
- Free in gluten—so used for wheat food allergy and celiac disease.
- Rich in riboflavin, niacin, thiamin, pantothenic acid, vitamin B_6, and folic acid which works as a co-factors for cellular substrate metabolism.

RAISIN

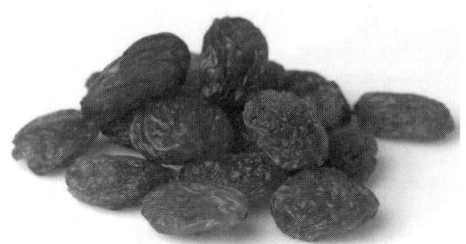

(Per 100 gm)			
Energy	299 kcal	Carbohydrates	79.18 g
Protein	3.07 g	Fat	0.46 g
Cholesterol	0 mg	Dietary fiber	3.7 g
Potassium	749 mg	Calcium	50 mg
Copper	0.318 mg	Iron	1.88 mg
Magnesium	7 mg	Manganese	0.299 mg
Phosphorus	101 mg	Selenium	0.6 µg
Zinc	0.22 mg	Folic acid	5 µg
Niacin	0.766 mg	Pantothenic acid	0.095 mg
Pyridoxine	0.0174 mg	Riboflavin	0.125 mg
Thiamin	0.106 mg	Vitamin A	0 IU
Vitamin C	2.3 mg	Vitamin E	0.12 mg
Vitamin K	3.5 µg		

- Very rich in energy.
- Contains phytochemical compound resveratrol—polyphenol anti-oxidant which has anti-inflammatory, anti-malignancy, blood cholesterol lowering property so helpful in preventing coronary heart disease, stroke, degenerative nerve disease and Alzheimer's disease.
- Rich in thiamin, pyridoxine, riboflavin and pantothenic acid.
- High in anthocyanins—antioxidants acts as anti-allergic, anti-inflammatory, anti-microbial and anti-malignancy.
- Rich in flavonoid such as tartaric acid, tannins and catechins.
- Rich in potassium which is helpful in controlling heart rate and blood pressure.

- Free of gluten.
- Rich in calcium, iron, manganese, magnesium copper, fluoride and zinc.

CASHEW NUT

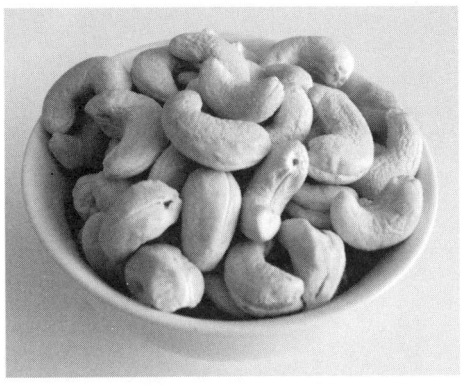

"heart-friendly"

(Per 100 gm)			
Energy	553 kcal	Carbohydrates	30.19 g
Protein	18.22 g	Fat	43.85 g
Cholesterol	0 mg	Dietary fiber	3.3 g
Sodium	12 mg	Potassium	660 mg
Calcium	37 mg	Copper	2.195 mg
Iron	6.68 mg	Magnesium	292 mg
Manganese	1.655 mg	Phosphorus	593 mg
Selenium	19.9 µg	Zinc	5.78 mg
Folic acid	25 µg	Niacin	1.062 mg
Pantothenic acid	0.864 mg	Pyridoxine	0.417 mg
Riboflavin	0.058 mg	Thiamin	0.423 mg
Vitamin A	0 IU	Vitamin C	0.5 mg
Vitamin E	5.31 mg	Vitamin K	4.1 µg

- Very high in calories.
- Rich in pantothenic acid, pyridoxine, riboflavin, and thiamin.
- Contains zeaxanthin pigment flavonoid antioxidant, which prevents age-related macular degeneration.

- Rich in monounsaturated fatty acids like oleic, and palmitoleic acids. These essential fatty acids help lower LDL cholesterol and increasing HDL cholesterol. These prevent coronary artery disease and strokes.
- Rich source of manganese, potassium, copper, iron, magnesium, zinc and selenium.

DATES (Dry)

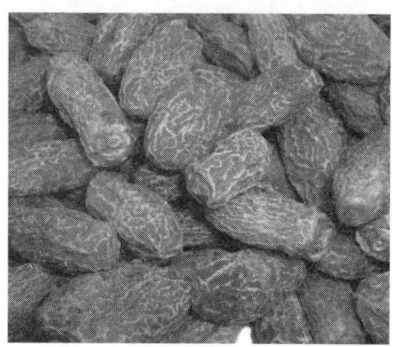

(Per 100 gm)			
Energy	277 kcal	Carbohydrates	74.97 g
Protein	1.81 g	Fat	0.15 g
Cholesterol	0 mg	Dietary fiber	6.7 g
Sodium	1 mg	Potassium	696 mg
Calcium	64 mg	Copper	0.362 mg
Iron	0.90 mg	Magnesium	54 mg
Manganese	0.296 mg	Phosphorus	62 mg
Zinc	0.44 mg	Folic acid	15 µg
Niacin	1.610 mg	Pantothenic acid	0.805 mg
Pyridoxine	0.249 mg	Riboflavin	0.060 mg
Thiamin	0.050 mg	Vitamin A	149 IU
Vitamin C	0 mg	Vitamin K	2.7 µg

- Contains simple sugars—fructose and dextrose.
- Rich in dietary fiber, which prevents LDL cholesterol and also acts as bulk laxative.
- Contains antioxidant flavonoid such as β-carotene, lutein, and zeaxanthin which protects from colon, prostate, breast, endometrial, lung and pancreatic malignancies.

- Contains zeaxanthin dietary carotenoid which protects against age-related macular degeneration.
- Contains flavonoid polyphenolic antioxidants—tannins which is anti-infective, anti-inflammatory and anti-hemorrhagic.
- Rich in vitamin A which gives protection against lung and oral cavity malignancies.
- Rich in calcium, manganese, copper and magnesium.
- Excellent source of iron.
- Very good in potassium which controls heart rate and blood pressure.
- Contains adequate levels of B-complex group of vitamins as well as vitamin K.

OLIVE

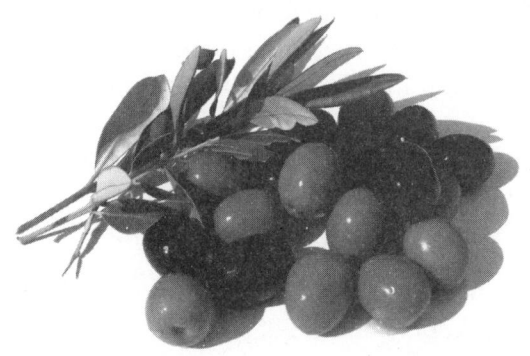

(Per 100 gm)			
Vitamin A	20 µg	Thiamine	0.021 mg
Riboflavin	0.007 mg	Niacin	0.237 mg
Vitamin B$_6$	0.031 mg	Folic acid	3 µg
Choline	14.2 mg	Vitamin E	3.81 mg
Vitamin K	1.4 µg	Energy	146 kcal
Carbohydrates	3.84 g	Sugars	0.54 g
Dietary fiber	3.3 g	Fat	15.32 g
Saturated	2.029 g	Monounsaturated	11.314 g
Polyunsaturated	1.307 g	Protein	1.03 g
Calcium	52 mg	Iron	0.49 mg
Magnesium	11 mg	Phosphorus	4 mg
Potassium	42 mg	Sodium	1556 mg

ARTICHOKES

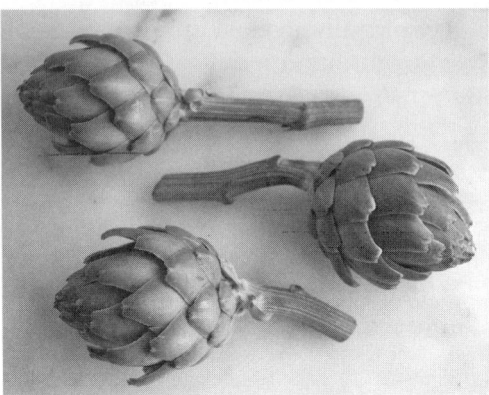

- Have highest antioxidant levels.
- Reduces chance of developing malignancy.
- Rich in magnesium, phosphorous, and manganese.
- Keeps brain healthy.
- Reduces the levels of bad cholesterol and increase the levels of good cholesterol.
- Rich in potassium which reduces blood pressure and heart diseases.
- Rich in dietary fiber which prevents constipation, stomach and intestinal malignancies.

BAEL (Aegle Marmelos)

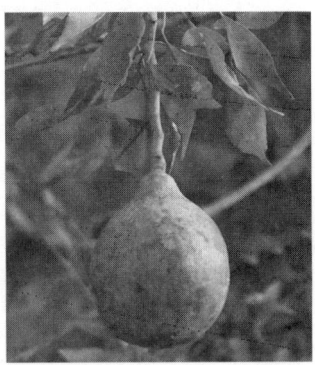

- In Hinduism the tree is sacred.
- Used in the worship of Shiva.
- Tri-foliate form of leaves symbolize the trident that Shiva holds in his right hand.
- Essential oil present in bael is effective against 21 types of bacteria.
- Prevention of constipation and other gastrointestinal problems.
- Prevents from giardia and rotavirus.

WALNUTS (Akrod)

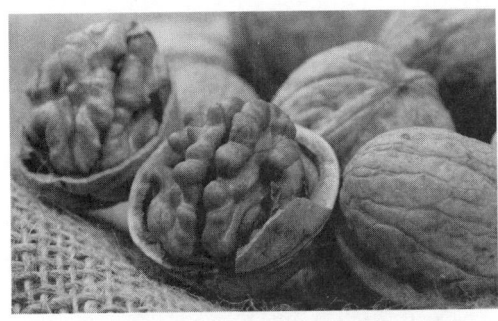

Energy	654 kcal	Carbohydrates	13.71 g
Protein	15.23 g	Fat	65.21 g
Cholesterol	0 mg	Dietary fiber	6.7 g
Sodium	2 mg	Potassium	441 mg
Calcium	98 mg	Copper	1.5 mg
Iron	2.9 mg	Magnesium	158 mg
Manganese	3.4 mg	Phosphorus	346 mg
Selenium	4.9 µg	Zinc	3.09 mg
Folic acid	98 µg	Niacin	1.125 mg
Pantothenic acid	0.570 mg	Pyridoxine	0.537 mg
Riboflavin	0.150 mg	Thiamin	0.341 mg
Vitamin A	20 IU	Vitamin C	1.3 mg
Vitamin E	20.83 mg	Vitamin K	2.7 µg

- Rich source of energy.
- Rich in monounsaturated fatty acids—omega-3 essential fatty acids like linoleic acid, alpha-linolenic acid (ALA) and arachidonic acids.

- Rich in riboflavin, niacin, thiamin, pantothenic acid, vitamin B_6, and folic acid.
- Rich in manganese, copper, potassium, calcium, iron, magnesium, zinc, and selenium.
- Oil used in massage therapy, aromatherapy, in pharmaceutical and cosmetic industries.
- Helps to lower total as well as LDL cholesterol and increases HDL cholesterol levels in the blood.
- Helps to lower blood pressure.
- Prevents coronary artery disease, strokes and breast, colon and prostate malignancies.
- Rich in melatonin, ellagic acid, vitamin E, carotenoids, and polyphenolic compounds. These prevent malignancy, aging, inflammation, and neurological diseases.

DRIED FIGS

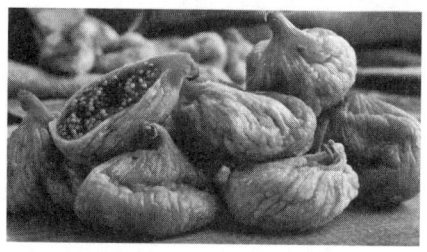

(1 Fig.)			
Energy	47 kcal	Protein	0.63 g
Fat	0.18 g	Carbohydrate	12.14 g
Fiber	0.9 g	Sugars	9.1 g
Calcium, Ca	31 mg	Iron, Fe	0.39 mg
Magnesium, Mg	13 mg	Phosphorus, P	13 mg
Potassium, K	129 mg	Sodium, Na	2 mg
Zinc, Zn	0.1 mg	Copper, Cu	0.055 mg
Thiamin	0.016 mg	Riboflavin	0.016 mg
Niacin	0.118 mg	Folic acid, total	2 mcg
Vitamin A	2 IU	Vitamin E	0.07 mg
Vitamin K	3 mcg		

- Rich in potassium have role in controlling blood pressure.
- Rich in dietary fiber.
- Contains tryptophan which induces good sleep.
- Relieves fatigue and boosts memory power.
- For curing hemorrhoids or piles.
- Reduces the risk of breast malignancy.
- Rich in calcium and potassium which prevents bone thinning and promotes bone density.

POMEGRANATE

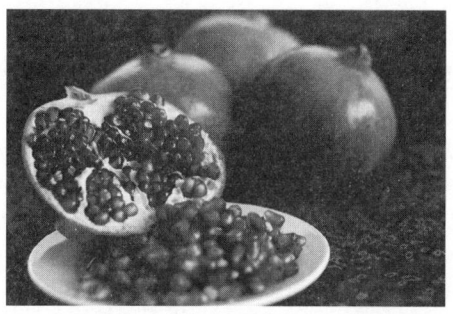

(Per 100 gm)			
Energy	83 kcal	Carbohydrates	18.70 g
Protein	1.67 g	Fat	1.17 g
Cholesterol	0 mg	Dietary fiber	4 g
Electrolytes		Sodium	3 mg
Potassium	236 mg	Calcium	10 mg
Copper	18%	Iron	0.30 mg
Magnesium	12 mg	Manganese	0.119 mg
Phosphorus	36 mg	Selenium	0.5 µg
Zinc	0.35 mg	Folic acid	38 µg
Niacin	0.293 mg	Pantothenic acid	0.135 mg
Pyridoxine	0.075 mg	Riboflavin	0.053 mg
Thiamin	0.067 mg	Vitamin A	0 IU
Vitamin C	10.2 mg	Vitamin E	0.60 mg
Vitamin K	16.4 µg		

- Moderate in calories.
- No cholesterol or saturated fats.
- Rich in soluble and insoluble dietary fibers.
- Good for weight reduction and cholesterol control.
- Good source of pantothenic acid (vitamin B_5), folic acid, pyridoxine and vitamin K.
- Rich in calcium, copper, potassium, and manganese.
- Boost up immunity, improves circulation, and offers protection from malignancies.
- Contains granatin B and punicalagin which reduces risk of heart diseases.
- Good source of antioxidant vitamin C.
- Protects against prostate malignancy, benign prostatic hyperplasia (BPH), diabetes, and lymphoma.

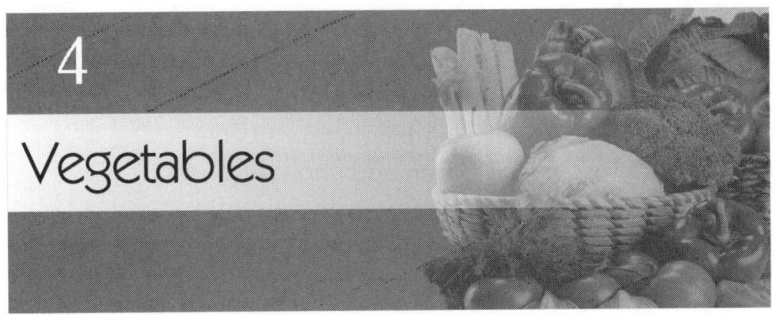

4

Vegetables

AMARNATH

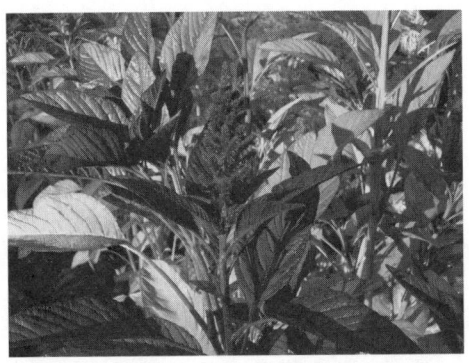

	(100 mg)		
Calorie	23	Fat	0.3 g
Saturated fat	0.1 gm	Cholesterol	0 mg
Sodium	20 mg	Carbohydrateohydrate	4 gm
Protein	2.5 g	Calcium	215.00 mg
Copper	0.162 mg	Iron	2.32 mg
Magnesium	55.00 mg	Manganese	0.885 mg
Phosphorus	50.00 mg	Potassium	611.00 mg
Selenium	0.9 mcg	Sodium	20.00 mg
Zinc	0.90 mg	Folic acid	85.00 mcg
Niacin	0.658 mg	Pantothenic acid	0.064 mg
Riboflavin	0.158 mg	Thiamin	0.027 mg
Vitamin A	146.00 mcg	Vitamin B$_6$	0.192 mg
Vitamin C	43.3 mg	Vitamin K	1140.0 mcg

- Rich in vitamins A, B, E and folic acid and vitamin C.
- Contains calcium, potassium, phosphorus, magnesium and zinc.
- Rich in vitamin C which boost up immunity.
- Keeps your hair black.
- Contains the oxalic acid which is helpful in absorbing the minerals like zinc and calcium.
- Rich in proteins.
- High fiber and essential amino acids which prevents the malignancy and controls cholesterol level in the body.
- Easily digestive food.

CABBAGE

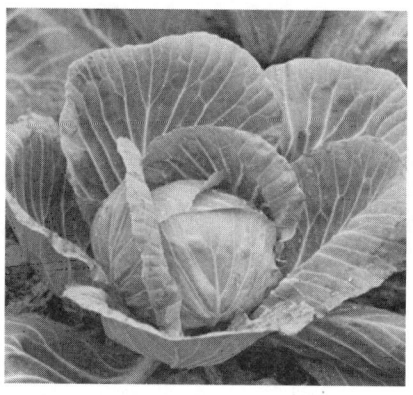

(Per 100 gm)			
Energy	25 kcal	Carbohydrates	5.8 g
Protein	1.3 g	Fat	0.1 g
Cholesterol	0 mg	Dietary fiber	2.50 mg
Folic acid	53 µg	Niacin	0.234 mg
Pantothenic acid	0.212 mg	Pyridoxine	0.124 mg
Riboflavin	0.040 mg	Thiamin	0.061 mg
Vitamin A	98 IU	Vitamin C	36.6 mg
Vitamin K	76 µg	Sodium	18 mg
Potassium	170 mg	Calcium	40 mg
Iron	0.47 mg	Magnesium	12 mg
Manganese	0.160 mg	Phosphorus	26 mg
Zinc	0.18 mg		

- Highly nutritious.
- Rich in phyto-chemicals like thiocyanates, indole-3-carbinol, lutein, zeaxanthin, sulforaphane, and isothiocyanates. These are powerful antioxidants which gives rise protection against breast, colon, and prostate malignancies and also reduces bad cholesterol in the blood.
- Rich in potassium, manganese, iron, and magnesium.
- Good source of vitamin K which has role in curing Alzheimer's disease.
- Rich in natural antioxidant—vitamin C which gives resistance against infectious agents and inflammatory free radicals.
- Rich in pantothenic acid 5, pyridoxine and thiamin.

CAULIFLOWER

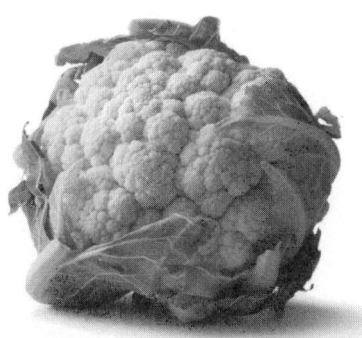

	(Per 100 gm)		
Energy	25 kcal	Carbohydrates	4.97 g
Protein	1.92 g	Fat	0.28 g
Cholesterol	0 mg	Dietary fiber	2.0 g
Folic acid	57 µg	Niacin	0.507 mg
Pantothenic acid	0.667 mg	Pyridoxine	0.184 mg
Riboflavin	0.060 mg	Thiamin	0.050 mg
Vitamin A	0 IU	Vitamin C	48.2 mg
Vitamin E	0.08 mg	Vitamin K	15.5 µg
Sodium	30 mg	Potassium	299 mg
Calcium	22 mg	Copper	0.039 mg
Iron	0.42 mg	Magnesium	15 mg
Manganese	0.155 mg	Zinc	0.27 mg

- Low in calories.
- Low in fat and no cholesterol.
- Contains anti-malignancy phyto-chemicals like sulforaphane and plant sterols such as indole-3-carbinol which has benefits against prostate, breast, cervical, colon, ovarian malignancies.
- Contains good amount of folic acid, pantothenic acid, pyridoxine and thiamin, niacin and vitamin K. These required for fat, protein and carbohydrate metabolism.
- Good source of manganese, copper, iron, calcium and potassium.
- Contains Di-indolyl-methane—a lipid soluble compound useful in the treatment of recurring respiratory papillomatosis caused by the Human Papillomavirus (HPV) and cervical dysplasia.
- Rich in vitamin C which boosts immunity and protects from malignancies.

FENUGREEK LEAVES (Methi)

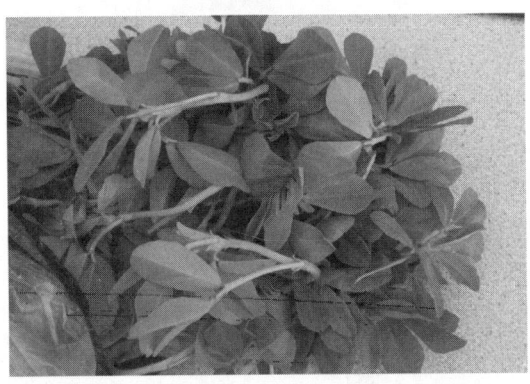

	(100 gm)		
Energy	49 kcals	Moisture	86 gm
Protein	4 gm	Fat	1 gm
Mineral	1 gm		
Rich in potassium, calcium and iron			
Rich in vitamin C			
Good amount of vitamin K			

- Leaves are cool and mildly laxative
- Helpful in digestion
- Useful in type-1 and type-2 diabetes.
- Lower serum cholesterol, triglyceride, and low-density lipoprotein.
- Prevent mouth ulcers.
- Good remedy for sore throat.
- Increases milk secretion in lactating mothers.
- Protect against breast and colon malignancies.

BROCCOLI

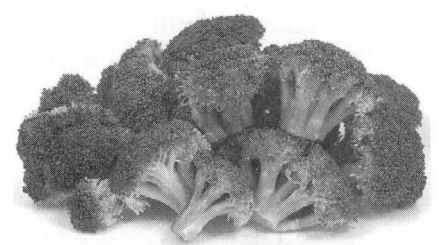

(Per 100 gm)			
Energy	34 kcal	Carbohydrates	6.64 g
Protein	2.82 g	Fat	0.37 g
Cholesterol	0 mg	Dietary fiber	2.60 g
Sodium	33 mg	Potassium	316 mg
Calcium	47 mg	Copper	0.049 mg
Iron	0.73 mg	Magnesium	21 mg
Manganese	0.210 mg	Selenium	2.5 µg
Zinc	0.41 mg	Folic acid	63 µg
Niacin	0.639 mg	Pantothenic acid	0.573 mg
Pyridoxine	0.175 mg	Riboflavin	0.117 mg
Thiamin	0.071 mg	Vitamin A	623 IU
Vitamin C	89.2 mg	Vitamin E	0.17 mg
Vitamin K	101.6 µg		

- Very low calorie vegetables.
- Contains many phyto-nutrients such as thiocyanates, indoles, sulforaphane, isothiocyanates.

- Good source of flavonoids like beta-carotene cryptoxanthin, lutein, and zeaxanthin.
- Excellent source of folic acid which prevent neural tube defects in the offspring.
- Rich source of vitamin K, niacin, pantothenic acid, pyridoxine and riboflavin.
- Good source of calcium, manganese, iron, magnesium, selenium, zinc and phosphorus.
- Gives protection from prostate, colon, urinary bladder, pancreatic, and breast malignancies.
- Rich source of vitamin C—a powerful natural antioxidant and immune modulator.
- Good amount of vitamin A with pro-vitamins like beta-carotene, alpha-carotene, and zeaxanthin. These protects from macular degeneration of the retina.

SPINACH

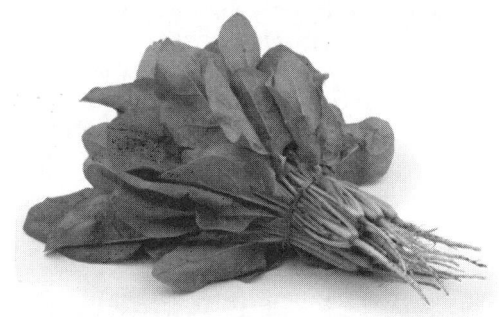

(Per 100 gm)			
Energy	23 kcal	Carbohydrates	3.63 g
Protein	2.86 g	Fat	0.39 g
Cholesterol	0 mg	Dietary fiber	2.2 g
Sodium	79 mg	Potassium	558 mg
Calcium	99 mg	Copper	0.130 mg
Iron	2.71 mg	Magnesium	79 mg
Manganese	0.897 mg	Zinc	0.53 mg
Folic acid	194 µg	Niacin	0.724 mg

(contd.)

Pantothenic acid	0.065 mg	Pyridoxine	0.195 mg
Riboflavin	0.189 mg	Thiamin	0.078 mg
Vitamin A	9377 IU	Vitamin C	28.1 mg
Vitamin E	2.03 mg	Vitamin K	482.9 µg

- Low in calories and fats.
- Contains a good amount of soluble dietary fiber.
- Recommended for cholesterol controlling and weight reduction purpose.
- One of the iron rich green leafy vegetables.
- Rich source of vitamin C—powerful antioxidants.
- Good amount of potassium, manganese, magnesium, copper and zinc.
- Rich source of omega-3 fatty acids.
- Prevents osteoporosis and iron-deficiency anemia.
- Rich source of vitamin A, vitamin C, and flavonoid poly phenolic antioxidants such as lutein, zeaxanthin and beta-carotene.
- Contains zeaxanthin which protect from age-related macular disease.
- Protection from lung and oral cavity malignancies.
- Excellent source of vitamin K which has a role in Alzheimer's disease.
- Good source of pyridoxine, thiamin, riboflavin, folic acid and niacin.

RUTABAGA

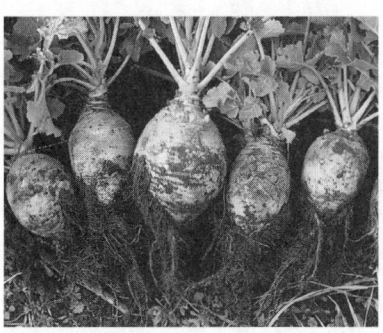

(Per 100 gm)			
Energy	38 kcal	Carbohydrates	8.62 g
Sugars	4.46 g	Dietary fiber	2.3 g
Fat	0.16 g	Protein	1.08 g
Vitamin C	25 mg	Calcium	43 mg
Iron	0.44 mg	Magnesium	20 mg
Manganese	0.131 mg	Phosphorus	53 mg
Potassium	305 mg	Zinc	0.24 mg
Thiamine	0.09 mg	Riboflavin	0.04 mg
Niacin	0.7 mg	Pantothenic acid	0.16 mg
Vitamin B_6	0.1 mg	Folic acid	21 µg

- Contains phytochemicals which inhibits the growth of malignant tumors.
- Good source of antioxidants which prevents free radical damage to DNA.
- High in potassium.
- Weight loss—low calorie and high nutrient content helps to regulate body weight.
- Rich in vitamin C—a powerful antioxidant known to boost the immune system.
- Good source of fiber.
- Glucosinolates present in rutabaga has a role in helicobacter pylori.

CORRIANDER LEAVES

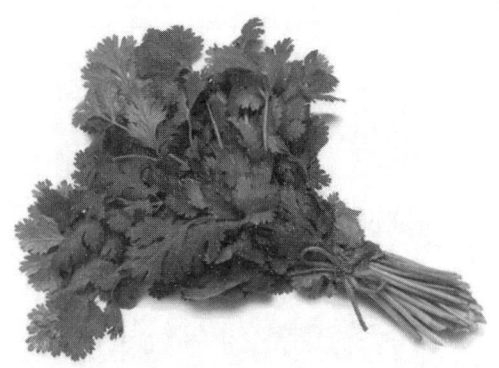

(Per 100 gm)			
Energy	23 kcal	Carbohydrates	3.67 g
Protein	2.13 g	Fat	0.52 g
Cholesterol	0 mg	Dietary fiber	2.80 g
Sodium	46 mg	Potassium	521 mg
Calcium	67 mg	Iron	1.77 mg
Magnesium	26 mg	Manganese	0.426 mg
Phosphorus	48 mg	Selenium	0.9 mg
Zinc	0.50 mg	Folic acid	62 µg
Niacin	1.114 mg	Pantothenic acid	0.570 mg
Pyridoxine	0.149 mg	Riboflavin	0.162 mg
Thiamin	0.067 mg	Vitamin A	6748 IU
Vitamin C	27 mg	Vitamin E	2.50 mg
Vitamin K	310 mcg		

- No cholesterol.
- Rich in antioxidants which help to reduce LDL.
- Contain many essential volatile oils such as borneol, linalool, cineole, cymene, terpineol, dipentene, phellandrene, pinene and terpinolene.
- Rich in antioxidant polyphenolic flavonoids such as quercetin, kaempferol, rhamnetin and epigenin.
- Traditional medicines such as analgesic, aphrodisiac, antispasmodic, deodorant, digestive, carminative, fungicidal, lipolytic, stimulant and stomachic.
- Antiseptic and carminative properties.
- Good source of potassium, calcium, manganese, iron, and magnesium.
- Rich in folic acid, riboflavin, niacin, vitamin A, beta carotene, vitamin C.
- Good source of vitamin A , which gives protection from lung and oral cavity malignancies.
- Richest herbal sources for vitamin K have role in the treatment of Alzheimer's disease.

CASSAVA (Topioca)

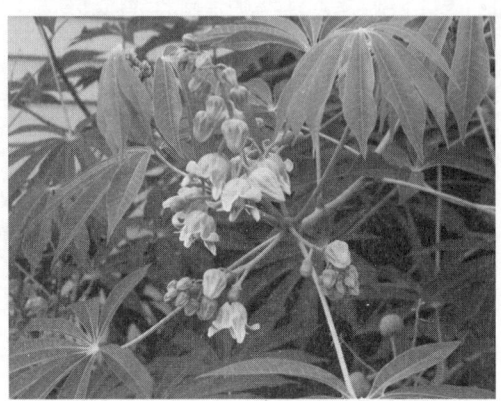

(Per 100 gm)			
Energy	670 cal	Protein	1.4 g
Fat	0.28 g	Carbohydrates	38 g
Fiber	1.8 g	Calcium	16 mg
Iron	0.27 mg	Magnesium	21 mg
Phosphorus	27 mg	Potassium	271 mg
Sodium	14 mg	Zinc	0.34 mg
Copper	0.10 mg	Manganese	0.38 mg
Selenium	0.7 µg	Vitamin C	20.6 mg
Thiamin	0.09 mg	Riboflavin	0.05 mg
Niacin	0.85 mg	Pantothenic acid	0.11 mg
Vitamin B_6	0.09 mg	Folic acid	27 µg
Vitamin A (IU)	13	Vitamin E	0.19 mg
Vitamin K	1.9 µg		

- Essentially a carbohydrate source.
- Low content of vitamins and minerals.
- Rich in calcium and vitamin C.
- Good source of thiamine, riboflavin and nicotinic acid.
- Poor source of protein.
- Had some antinutritional and toxic factors like cassava linamarin and lotaustralin. These, on hydrolysis, release hydrocyanic acid.

DRUMSTICK LEAVES

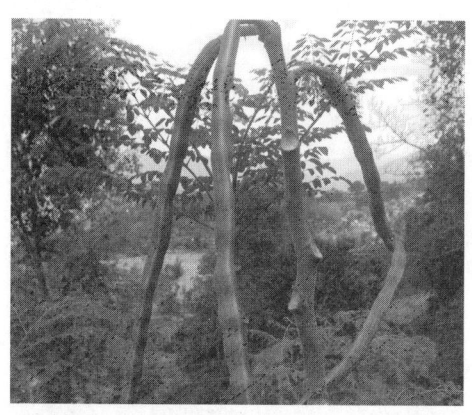

(Per serving)

Drumstick leaves:

Energy	64 kcal	Carbohydrates	8.2
Protein	9.40 g	Fat	1.40
Dietary Fiber	2.0 g	Sodium	9 mg
Potassium	337 mg	Calcium	185 mg
Iron	4.00 mg	Magnesium	147 mg
Phosphorus	112 mg	Selenium	0.9 µg
Zinc	0.60 mg	Folic acid	40 µg
Niacin	2.220 mg	Pyridoxine	1.200 mg
Riboflavin	0.660 mg	Thiamin	0.257 mg
Vitamin A	7564 IU	Vitamin C	51.7 mg

In pod-per serving:

Energy	37 kcal	Carbohydrates	8.53 g
Protein	2.10 g	Fat	0.20 g
Dietary fiber	3.2 g	Sodium	42 mg
Potassium	461 mg	Calcium	30 mg
Iron	0.36 mg	Magnesium	45 mg
Phosphorus	50 mg	Selenium	8.2 µg
Zinc	0.45 mg	Folic acid	44 µg
Niacin	0.680 mg	Pyridoxine	0.120 mg
Riboflavin	0.074 mg	Thiamin	0.053 mg
Vitamin A	74 IU	Vitamin C	141 mg

- Leaves are good source of protein.
- Fresh pods and seeds are rich in oleic acid, a health-benefiting monounsaturated fat.
- Richest source of vitamin A which maintenace skin integrity, vision and immunity.
- Excellent sources of vitamin C.
- Rich in folic acid, vitamin B$_6$, thiamin, riboflavin, pantothenic acid, and niacin.
- Sources of calcium, iron, copper, manganese, zinc, selenium, and magnesium.

LETTUCE

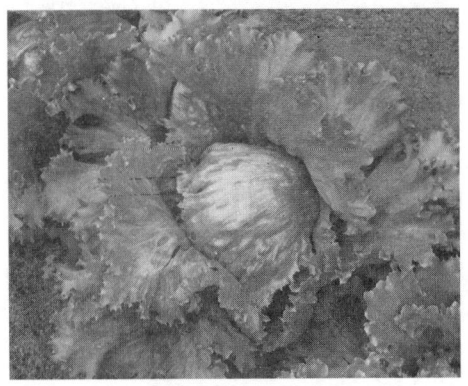

(Per 100 gm)			
Energy	15 kcal	Carbohydrates	2.79 g
Protein	1.36 g	Fat	0.15 g
Cholesterol	0 mg	Dietary Fiber	1.3 g
Sodium	28 mg	Potassium	194 mg
Calcium	36 mg	Copper	0.029 mg
Iron	0.86 mg	Magnesium	13 mg
Manganese	0.250 mg	Phosphorus	29 mg
Zinc	0.18 mg	Folic acid	38 µg
Niacin	0.375 mg	Pantothenic acid	0.134 mg
Pyridoxine	0.090 mg	Riboflavin	0.080 mg
Thiamin	0.070 mg	Vitamin A	7405 IU
Vitamin C	9.2 mg	Vitamin E	0.29 mg
Vitamin K	126.3 µg		

- Very low calorie green vegetables.
- Excellent source of several vitamin A and beta carotenes which are essential for vision.
- Rich in flavonoids that protects the body from lung and oral cavity malignancies.
- Rich in iron, calcium, magnesium, and potassium.
- Rich in thiamin, vitamin B$_6$ riboflavins.
- Prevents osteoporosis, iron-deficiency anemia, cardiovascular diseases, Alzheimer's disease and malignancies.
- Rich source of vitamin K which has role in Alzheimer's disease.
- Rich in folic acid and vitamin C.
- Contains zeaxanthin—dietary carotenoid gives protection against age-related macular disease.

THAI BASIL

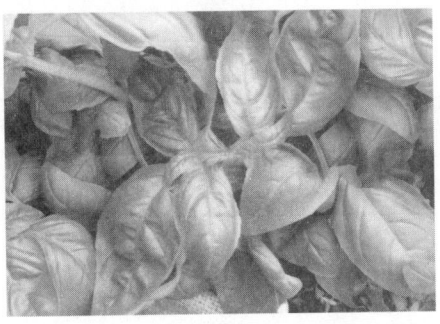

(Per 100 gm)			
Energy	22 kcal	Carbohydrates	2.65 g
Dietary fiber	1.6 g	Fat	0.64 g
Protein	3.15 g	Vitamin K	414.8 μg
Calcium	177 mg	Iron	3.17 mg
Magnesium	64 mg	Manganese	1.148 mg
Phosphorus	56 mg	Potassium	295 mg
Sodium	4 mg	Zinc	0.81 mg
Vitamin A	264 μg	Thiamine	0.034 mg
Riboflavin	0.076 mg	Niacin	0.902 mg
Pantothenic acid	0.209 mg	Vitamin B$_6$	0.155 mg
Folic acid	68 μg	Vitamin C	18.0 mg
Vitamin E	0.80 mg		

- Very low in calories.
- Contains stevioside—a non-carbohydrate glycoside compound which have long shelf life, high temperature tolerance, non-fermentative; but contain near-zero calories.
- Used to reduce weight.
- Basil oil has potent antioxidant, antiviral, and antimicrobial properties, and potential for use in treating.
- Contains many sterols and antioxidant compounds like triterpenes, flavonoids, and tannins. These reduce the risk of pancreatic malignancy.
- Help to lower blood pressure.
- Inhibits caries causing bacteria in the mouth.

KALE

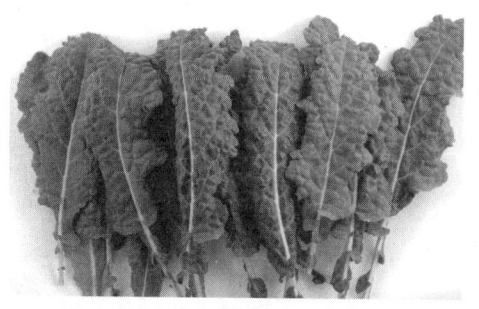

(Per 100 gm)			
Energy	49 calories	Carbohydrates	10.01 g
Protein	3.30 g	Fat	0.70 g
Cholesterol	0 mg	Dietary fiber	2.0 g
Sodium	43 mg	Potassium	447 mg
Calcium	135 mg	Copper	0.290 mg
Iron	1.70 mg	Magnesium	34 mg
Manganese	0.774 mg	Phosphorus	56 mg
Selenium	0.9 µg	Zinc	0.44 mg
Folic acid	29 µg	Niacin	1.000 mg
Pantothenic acid	0.091 mg	Pyridoxine	0.271 mg
Riboflavin	0.130 mg	Thiamin	0.110 mg
Vitamin A	15376 IU	Vitamin C	120 mg
Vitamin K	817 µg		

- Nutritious green leafy vegetable.
- Contains phytochemicals, sulforaphane and indole-3-carbinol which protect against prostate and colon malignancies.
- Contains di-indolyl-methane which is immune modulator, anti-bacterial and anti-viral.
- Good sources of vitamin-K having curative role in Alzheimer's disease.
- Rich in vitamin C—a powerful antioxidant, which helps against infectious agents.
- Good in niacin, vitamin B_6, thiamin and pantothenic acid.
- Rich in copper, calcium, sodium, potassium, iron, manganese, and phosphorus.
- Prevents osteoporosis, iron-deficiency anemia and malignancies of colon and prostate.
- Rich source of β-carotene, lutein and zeaxanthin. These flavonoids have antioxidant and antimalignancy activities.
- Contains zeaxanthin which gives protection against age-related macular degeneration.
- Rich in vitamin A which gives protection against lung and oral cavity malignancies.

LOTUS ROOT

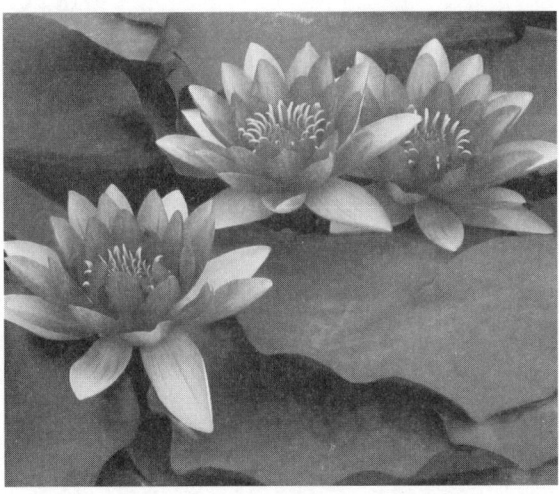

(Per 100 gm)			
Energy	74 kcal	Carbohydrates	17.23 g
Protein	2.60 g	Fat	0.10 g
Cholesterol	0 mg	Dietary fiber	4.9 g
Sodium	40 mg	Potassium	556 mg
Calcium	45 mg	Copper	0.257 mg
Iron	1.16 mg	Magnesium	23 mg
Manganese	0.261 mg	Selenium	0.7 µg
Zinc	0.39 mg	Folic acid	13 µg
Niacin	0.400 mg	Pantothenic acid	0.377 mg
Pyridoxine	0.258 mg	Riboflavin	0.220 mg
Thiamin	0.160 mg	Vitamin A	0 IU
Vitamin C	44 mg		

- Moderate calorie content.
- Good source dietary fibers which reduces blood cholesterol, sugar, body weight and relieves constipation.
- Rich in copper, iron, zinc, magnesium and manganese.
- Rich in potassium, so controls heart rate and blood pressure.
- Excellent sources of vitamin C—powerful water soluble antioxidant which is required for the collagen synthesis in the body.
- Also prevents scurvy, boosts up immunity and hasten wound healing.
- Rich in pyridoxine, folic acid, niacin, riboflavin, pantothenic acid, and thiamin. These have role in protection of heart attack by controlling harmful homocysteine levels in the blood.

CURRY LEAVES

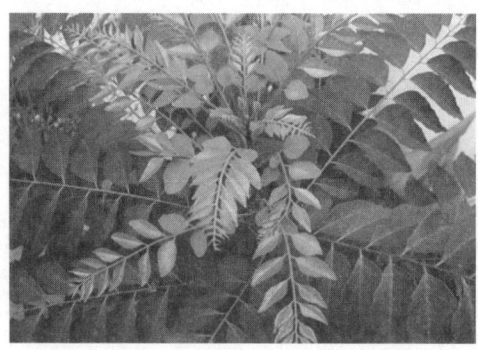

(Per 100 gm)			
Protein	6.1 gm	Fat	1 gm
Carbohydrates	18.7 gm	Fiber	4.2 gm
Calcium	830 mg	Vitamin A_{12}	600 IU
Phosphorus	57 mg	Iron	7 mg
Nicotinic acid	2.3 mg	Vitamin C	4 mg
Folic acid	23.500 µg	Thiamine	7560.000 µg
Magnesium	44.000 mg	Copper	0.100 mg
Zinc	0.200 mg		

- Rich in vitamin A, vitamin B, vitamin B_2, vitamin C, calcium and iron.
- Have anti-diabetic, antioxidant, antimicrobial and anti-inflammatory properties.
- Control diarrhea and dysentery.
- Reduces weight.
- Leucoderma.
- Anthelmintic and analgesic action.
- Reduce serum urea and creatinine.
- Herbal tonic.
- In the treatment of morning sickness, nausea and vomiting.
- Reduce total cholesterol and triglyceride levels.
- Improve eyesight and prevent cataract.
- Delays greying of hair.
- Improve appetite.
- Relieve nausea, heartburn and indigestion.
- Prevents obesity.
- Improves cognitive functions and reverses.
- Have anti-malignancy activity.
- Useful in type-2 diabetes by reducing sugar levels.

PARSLEY

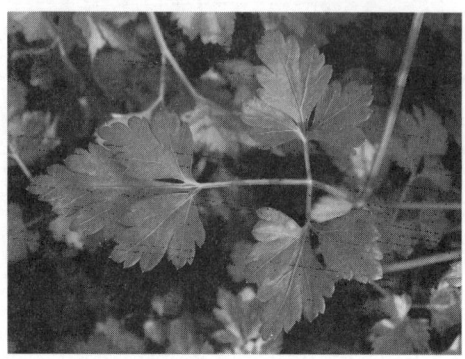

	(Per 100 gm)		
Energy	36 kcal	Carbohydrates	6.33 g
Dietary fiber	3.3 g	Fat	0.79 g
Protein	2.97 g	Calcium	138 mg
Iron	6.2 mg	Magnesium	50 mg
Manganese	0.16 mg	Phosphorus	58 mg
Potassium	554 mg	Sodium	56 mg
Zinc	1.07 mg	Vitamin A	421 µg
Thiamine	0.086 mg	Riboflavin	0.09 mg
Niacin	1.313 mg	Pantothenic acid	0.4 mg
Vitamin B_6	0.09 mg	Folic acid	152 µg
Vitamin C	133 mg	Vitamin E	0.75 mg
Vitamin K	1640 µg		

- Good source of antioxidants—luteolin, apigenin, folic acid, vitamins K, C and A.
- Excessive consumption should be avoided by pregnant women because of uterotonic effects.
- Adequate in vitamin K which has role in nervous system.
- Role in Anemia prevention
- Contains Myristicin which inhibits tumor formation in the lungs, also have a role in colon and prostate malignancy.
- Rich with an antioxidant arsenal
- Rich in vitamin C which have role in osteoarthritis and rheumatoid arthritis.

- Rich in folic acid which converts homocysteine into harmless molecules so decreases risk of heart attack, stroke and atherosclerosis.

CELERY

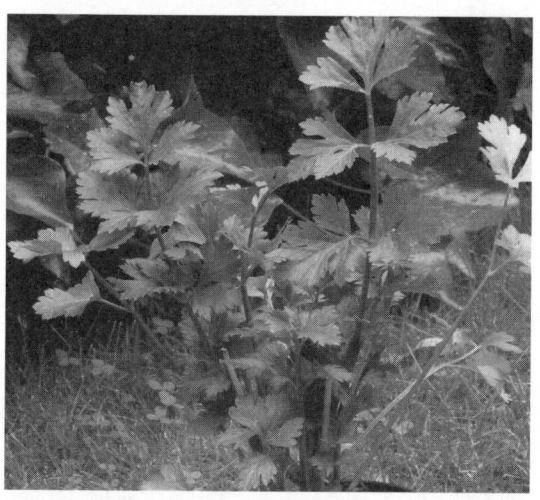

(Per 100 gm)			
Energy	16 kcal	Carbohydrates	3 g
Sugars	1.4 g	Dietary fibre	1.6 g
Fat	0.2 g	Protein	0.7 g
Calcium	40 mg	Iron	0.2 mg
Magnesium	11 mg	Phosphorus	24 mg
Potassium	260 mg	Sodium	80 mg
Zinc	0.13 mg	Vitamin A	22 µg
Thiamine	0.021 mg	Riboflavin	0.057 mg
Niacin	0.323 mg	Vitamin B_6	0.076 mg
Folic acid	36 µg	Vitamin C	3 mg
Vitamin E	0.27 mg	Vitamin K	29.3 µg

- Low calorie dietary fibre.
- Seeds contain 3-n-butylphthalide which controls blood pressure.

- Oil and seeds are uterine stimulant so avoided during pregnancy.
- Used in weight-loss diets.

ASAFOETIDA (Hing and Ting)

Food of the Gods

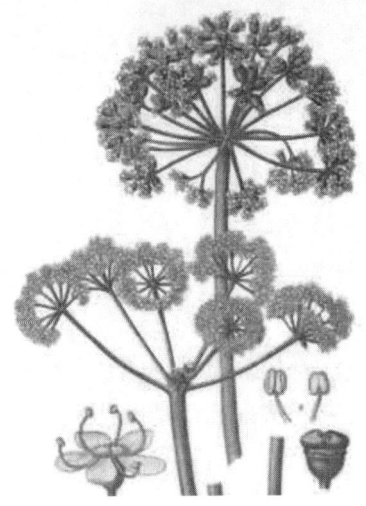

(Per 100 gm)			
Energry	297 cal	Moisture	16 gm
Protein	4 gm	Fat	1 gm
Mineral	7 gm	Fibre	4 gm
Carbohydrates	68 gm	Calcium	690 mg
Phosphorous	50 mg	Iron	39 mg

- Antiflatulent.
- Protects against influenza, asthma and bronchitis.
- It has property of contraceptive and abortifacient.
- It is antiepileptic.
- Helps in digestion.
- Balancing the vata and kapha.

AJWAIN SEEDS (Onva)

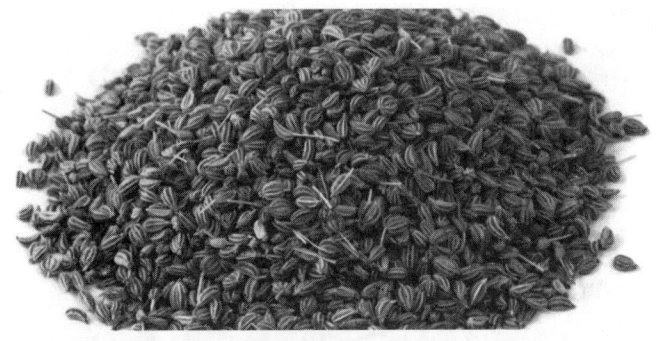

(Per 100 gm)			
Energy	305 calories	Fat	25 gm
Sodium	10 mg	Carbohydrates	43 gm
Dietary fiber	39 gm	Protein	16 gm

- Excellent source of essential oils—thymol, cymene, pinene, terpinene and limonene.
- Beneficial effect on digestive system.
- Curbs desire for drinking alcohol.
- Useful in infantile colic.
- Used in cases of diarrhea.
- Have anti-bacterial, germicide, antifungal and anesthetic properties.
- Rich in various vitamins, minerals, fibers and antioxidants.
- Home remedy for dyspepsia.
- Useful in ear infections and earache, arthritis.
- Useful in spasmodic pains due to indigestion and flatulence.
- Useful in acidity, migraine headache and common cold.
- Beneficial during pregnancy as it maintains the proper health of the uterus.

BETEL LEAF

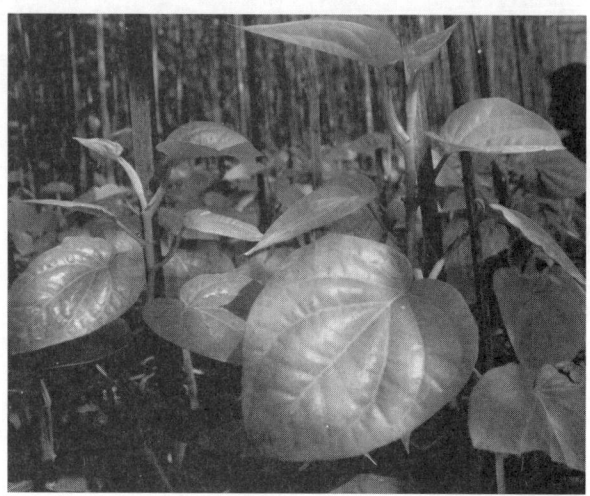

(Per 100 gm)			
Energy	44 cal	Moisture	85 gm
Protein	3 gm	Fat	1 gm
Mineral	2 gm	Fibre	2 gm
Carbohydrates	6 gm	Calcium	230 mg
Phosphorous	40 mg		

- Useful in treatment of bad breath, boils and abscesses, conjunctivitis, constipation, headache, hysteria, itches, mastitis, mastoiditis, leucorrhoea, otorrhoea, ringworm, swelling of gum, rheumatism, abrasion, cuts and injuries, etc.
- Leaves contain enzymes like diastase and catalase.
- Chewing of betel leaves produce a sense of well-being, increased alertness, sweating, salivation, hot sensation and energetic feeling with exhilaration.
- Root is used as female contraceptive.
- It is good appetizer, digestive, and refreshing mastication.
- Increases physical and mental functions.

POTATO

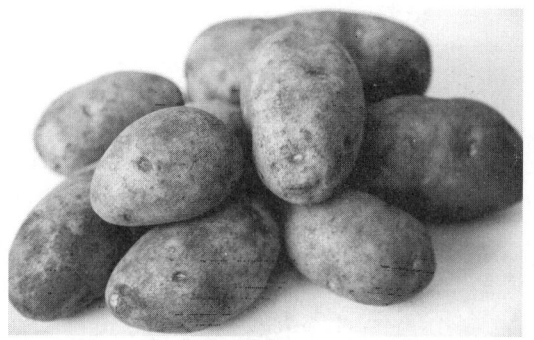

(Per 100 gm)			
Energy	70 kcal	Carbohydrates	15.9 g
Starch	15 g	Dietary fiber	2.5 g
Fat	0.1 g	Protein	1.89 g
Water	75 g	Vitamin B_3	1.05 mg
Vitamin B_5	0.3 mg	Vitamin B_6	0.3 mg
Vitamin C	11.4 mg	Calcium	10 mg
Iron	0.73 mg	Magnesium	22 mg
Phosphorus	61 mg	Potassium	455 mg

- Useful in diarrheal disorder cases.
- It is a players' diet because energy produced through potato gets stored as glycogen in muscle and readily available energy during prolonged, strenuous exercise.
- Increases brain function.
- Prevents kidney stones
- Keeps skin healthy.
- Rich in vitamin C, B_6, copper, manganese, and dietary fiber.
- Prevents heart attack and stroke.
- Raises the glucose level in the blood.
- May cause obesity.
- Reduces inflammation.

TOMATO

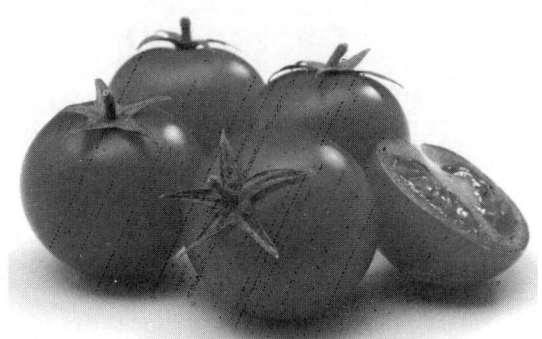

(Per 100 gm)			
Energy	18 kcal	Carbohydrates	3.9 g
Fat	0.2 g	Dietary fiber	1.2 g
Protein	0.9 g	Calcium	10 mg
Iron	0.3 mg	Magnesium	11 mg
Potassium	237 mg	Lycopene	2573 g
Vitamin A	833 IU	Vitamin B$_3$	0.59 mg
Vitamin E	0.54 mg	Vitamin C	13 mg

- Contains 'lycopene' pigment which is a vital antioxidant that protects against malignant cell formation.
- Rich source of vitamins and minerals.
- Contains high potassium that helps to maintain nerve health.
- Reduces the risk of malignancy.
- Reduces the risk of heart diseases.
- Prevents DNA damage.
- Protects against thrombosis.
- Reduces the inflammation.
- Also have high iron helps to maintain blood health.
- Rich in vitamin K which have role in blood clotting.
- Improves eye health.
- Prevents hypertension and urinary tract infections.

LADYFINGER (Okra)

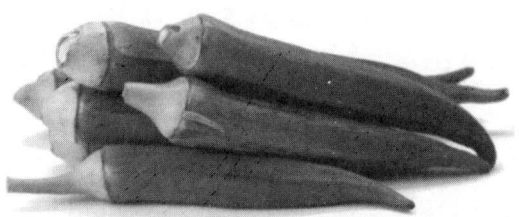

(Per 100 gm)			
Energy	33 kcal	Carbohydrates	7.45 g
Dietary fiber	3.2 g	Fat	0.19 g
Protein	2 g	Vitamin A	36 µg
Vitamin B$_3$	1 mg	Vitamin C	23 mg
Vitamin E	0.27 mg	Vitamin K	31.3 µg
Calcium	82 mg	Iron	0.62 mg
Magnesium	57 mg	Potassium	299 mg
Zinc	0.58 mg		

- Prevents diabetes.
- Reduces the neural tube defects in a newborn baby.
- Decreases absorption of cholesterol preventing heart diseases.
- Role in strengthening the bones in body.
- Prevents asthma, sun strokes, constipation, and colon malignancy.
- Avoids obesity.

CUCUMBER

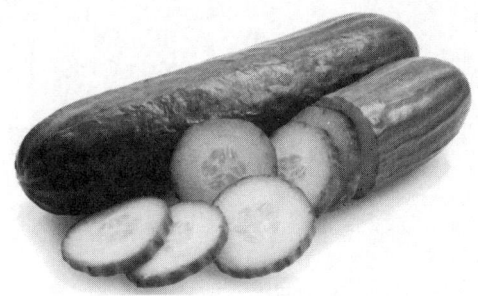

(Per 100 gm)			
Energy	16 kcal	Dietary fiber	0.5 g
Fat	0.11 g	Protein	0.65 g
Water	95.23 g	Vitamin B_5	0.3 mg
Folic acid	7 µg	Vitamin C	2.8 mg
Vitamin K	16.4 µg	Calcium	16 mg
Iron	0.28 mg	Magnesium	13 mg
Phosphorus	24 mg	Potassium	147 mg
Sodium	2 mg		

- Rehydrates body that helps in removal of toxins from body.
- Used for skin irritation, sun burns and gives cooling effects to eyes.
- Helps in digestion and weight loss.
- Cures diabetes, reduces cholesterol.
- Controls blood pressure.
- Relieves gout and arthritic pain.
- Relieves bad breath of mouth.

CARROT

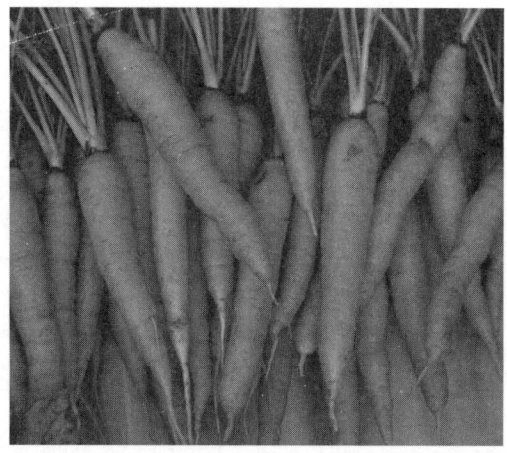

(Per 100 gm)			
Energy	27 kcal	Dietary fiber	2.3 g
Protein	0.59 g	Calcium	23 mg
Iron	0.27 mg	Magnesium	8 mg
Phosphorus	23 mg	Sodium	5 mg
Potassium	183 mg	Zinc	0.3 mg
Selenium	0.2 µg	Vitamin A	13286 IU
Vitamin B_3	0.5 mg	Vitamin B_5	0.12 mg
Vitamin B_9	11 µg	Vitamin E	0.8 mg
Vitamin K	10.7 µg		

- Improves vision and gives protection against senile cataract and macular degeneration.
- Keeps skin healthy and beautiful.
- Prevents heart diseases and strokes.
- Keeps teeth and gums healthy.
- Contains falcarinol and falcarindiol which acts as anti-malignancy, reduces risk of lung, breast and colon malignancy.
- Contains high levels of β-carotene which slows down the aging of cells.

RADDISH

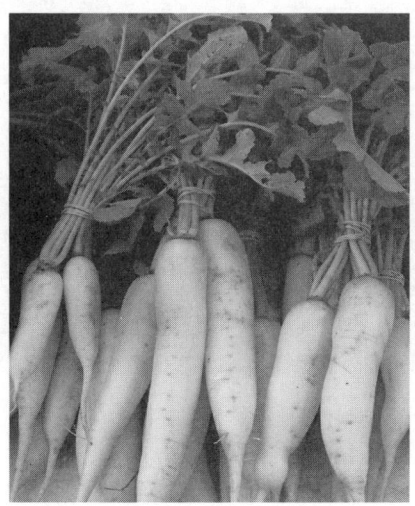

(Per 100 gm)			
Energy	16 kcal	Carbohydrates	3.4 g
Sugars	1.86 gm	Dietary fiber	1.6 g
Fat	0.1 g	Protein	0.68 g
Calcium	25 mg	Iron	0.34 mg
Magnesium	10 mg	Phosphorus	20 mg
Potassium	233 mg	Zinc	0.28 mg
Fluoride	6 µg	Vitamin B$_3$	0.254 mg
Vitamin B$_5$	0.165 mg	Vitamin B$_9$	25 µg
Vitamin C	14.8 mg		

- Low calories, high nutrients.
- Natures cooling food for summers.
- Soothens sore throat.
- Eliminates toxins and malignancy keeps hydrated.
- Fights cold and sinus block.
- Relieves indigestion.
- Prevents viral infections.

BEET

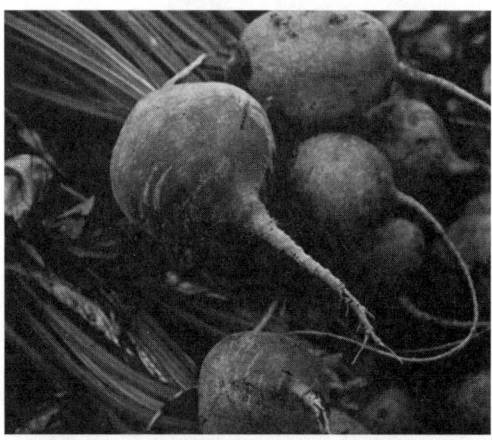

- High in carbohydrates.
- Rich in folic acid.
- Protects against heart disease.

(Per 100 gm)			
Energy	43 kcal	Carbohydrates	9.96 g
Dietary fiber	2 g	Fat	0.18 g
Protein	1.68 g	Calcium	16 mg
Iron	0.79 mg	Magnesium	23 mg
Phosphorus	38 mg	Sodium	77 mg
Potassium	308 mg	Zinc	0.35 mg
Vitamin B_3	0.33 mg	Vitamin B_5	0.15 mg
Vitamin B_6	0.067 mg	Vitamin B_9	80 µg
Vitamin C	3.6 mg		

- Fights against colon malignancy
- Contains betacyanin—pigment that gives red color which is anticarcinogenic.
- Strengthen the gall bladder and liver.

CHILI

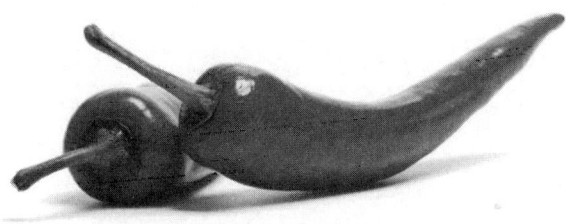

(Per 100 gm)			
Energy	40 kcal	Carbohydrates	8.8 g
Dietary fiber	1.5 g	Fat	0.4 g
Protein	1.9 g	Calcium	10 mg
Iron	1 mg	Magnesium	23 mg
Phosphorus	61 mg	Potassium	322 mg
Vitamin A	48 µg	Vitamin B_6	0.51 mg
Vitamin C	144 mg		

- Useful as analgesic in arthritis, diabetic neuropathy, post mastectomy pain, and headaches.
- Rich source of vitamin C.
- Helps in the process of digestion.

CAPSICUM

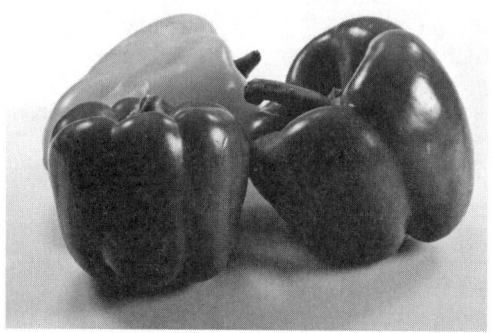

(Per 100 gm)			
Energy	40 kcal	Carbohydrates	9 g
Dietary fiber	1.5 g	Fat	0.2 g
Protein	2 g	Water	86 g
Vitamin B_6	0.51 mg	Vitamin C	144 mg
Vitamin E	0.58 mg	Calcium	10 mg
Iron	1 mg	Magnesium	23 mg
Phosphorus	61 mg	Potassium	340 mg
Capsaicin	1 mg		

- Plenty of vitamins C.
- Contains carotenoids (beta-carotene) which act as an anti-oxidant and anti-inflammatory.
- Reduces 'bad' cholesterol, controls diabetes, brings relief from pain and reduces inflammation.
- Have protective role in malignancies.
- Good source of vitamin E which keeps skin and hair healthy.
- Contains enzymes-lutein which protects eyes from cataracts and macular degeneration.
- Rich in vitamin B_6 which is essential for the health of the nervous system and helps renew cells.

BRINJAL

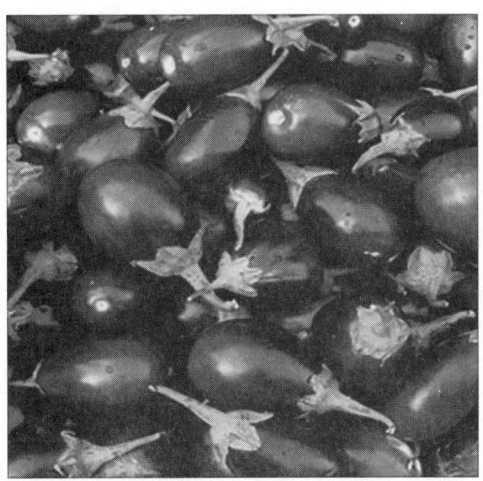

(Per 100 gm)			
Energy	25 kcal	Carbohydrates	5.88 g
Dietary fiber	3 g	Fat	0.18 g
Protein	0.98 g	Calcium	9 mg
Iron	0.23 mg	Magnesium	14 mg
Phosphorus	24 mg	Potassium	229 mg
Zinc	0.16 mg	Vitamin B_3	0.65 mg
Vitamin B_5	0.28 mg	Vitamin B_9	22 µg
Vitamin C	2.2 mg	Vitamin E	0.3 mg
Vitamin K	3.5 µg		

- Improves blood circulation and nourishes the brain.
- Protects from colon malignancy.
- High in bioflavonoids, which controls high blood pressure and relieve stress.
- Prevents blood clots due to presence of vitamin K and bioflavonoids, which strengthen capillaries.
- Used for controlling and managing diabetes due to high fiber and low soluble carbohydrate content.
- Lowers 'bad' cholesterol.

GARLIC

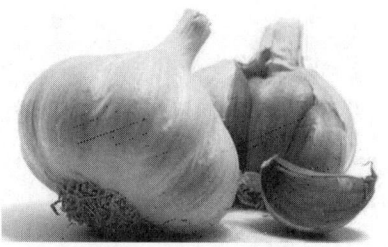

(Per 100 gm)			
Energy	149 kcal	Carbohydrates	33.06 g
Dietary fiber	2.1 g	Fat	0.5 g
Protein	6.36 g	Calcium	181 mg
Iron	1.7 mg	Magnesium	25 mg
Phosphorus	153 mg	Potassium	401 mg
Zinc	1.16 mg	Selenium	14.2 µg
Vitamin B_1	0.2 mg	Vitamin B_3	0.7 mg
Vitamin B_5	0.6 mg	Vitamin B_6	1.24 mg
Vitamin B_9	3 µg	Vitamin C	31.2 mg

- Useful in intrauterine life for weight gain of baby.
- Boosts up immune system.
- Prevents bladder, prostate, breast malignancy, colon, stomach malignancy.
- Prevents scurvy, fungal and bacterial vaginal infections.
- Lowers LDL cholesterol.

ONION

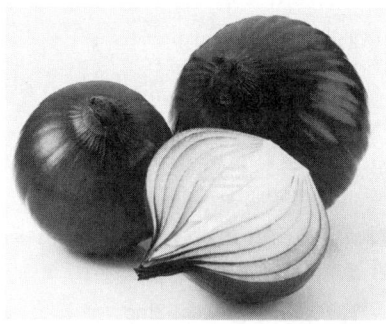

(Per 100 gm)			
Energy	40 kcal	Carbohydrates	9.34 g
Dietary fiber	1.7 g	Fat	0.1 g
Protein	1.1 g	Calcium	23 mg
Iron	0.21 mg	Magnesium	10 mg
Phosphorus	29 mg	Potassium	146 mg
Zinc	0.17 mg	Fluoride	1.1 µg
Vitamin B_3	0.116 mg	Vitamin B_5	0.123 mg
Vitamin B_6	0.12 mg	Vitamin B_9	19 µg
Vitamin C	7.4 mg		

- Offers protection against head and neck malignancy.
- Increases HDL (good) cholesterol production.
- Reduces osteoporosis.
- Increases insulin production.
- In case of honey bee bite—apply juice gives relief from pain.
- Reduces risk of developing gastric ulcers.
- Good remedy for insomnia, bleeding nose and flatulence.

MUSHROOM

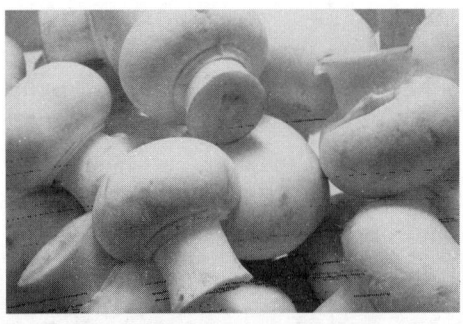

(Per 100 gm)			
Energy	27 kcal	Carbohydrates	4.1 g
Fat	0.1 g	Protein	2.5 g
Thiamine	0.1 mg	Riboflavin	0.5 mg
Niacin	3.8 mg	Pantothenic acid	1.5 mg
Vitamin C	0 mg	Calcium	18 mg
Phosphorus	120 mg	Potassium	448 mg
Sodium	6 mg	Zinc	1.1 mg

- Fleshy and edible fruit.
- Rich in water.
- Very low in calories.
- No cholesterol or fat.
- Very little sodium and fat.
- Ideal diet for hypertensive patients.
- Excellent source of potassium which lowers elevated blood pressure and reduces the risk of stroke.
- Rich source of riboflavin, niacin, and selenium.
- Decreases risk of prostate because of high selenium.
- White button mushrooms can reduce the risk of breast malignancy and prostate malignancy.
- Increased levels of potassium improve memory and knowledge retention.
- Rich in copper, calcium iron and selenium.
- Rich in fiber which helps to lower cholesterol levels.
- Good source of iron.
- Ideal low-energy diet for diabetics.
- Rich source of calcium.
- Rich in ergothioneine—a powerful antioxidant effective in boosting the immune system.
- Mushrooms contains natural antibiotics—similar to penicillin which inhibit microbial growth and other fungal infections.

BOTTLE GOURD (Lauki)

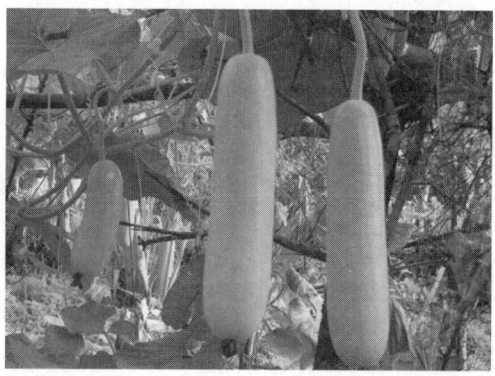

(Per 100 gm)			
Energy	15 kcal	Carbohydrates	3.69 g
Dietary fiber	1.2 g	Fat	0.02 g
Protein	0.6 g	Calcium	24 mg
Iron	0.25 mg	Magnesium	11 mg
Manganese	0.066 mg	Phosphorus	13 mg
Potassium	170 mg	Sodium	2 mg
Zinc	0.7 mg	Thiamine	0.029 mg
Riboflavin	0.022 mg	Niacin	0.39 mg
Pantothenic acid	0.144 mg	Vitamin B_6	0.038 mg
Folic acid	4 µg	Vitamin C	8.5 µg

- High in water content and fiber.
- Low in calories and fat.
- Natural diuretic.
- Easy to digest.
- Gives a cooling effect.
- Helpful for the diabetics and heart patients.
- Rich in iron, thiamine, magnesium, calcium and phosphorous.
- Low in sodium so useful for the hypertensive people.
- Useful in urinary burning.
- Used in jaundice.
- Rich in fiber so prevent constipation, flatulence and piles.
- Reduces the fatigue.

FRENCH BEANS

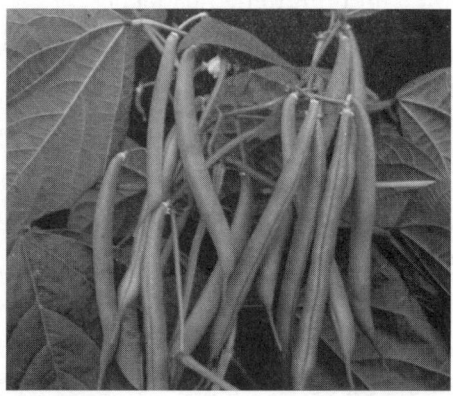

(1 cup)			
Energy	631 calories	Proteins	35 g
Carbohydrates	118 g	Dietary fiber	46 g
Fat	3.7 g	Calcium	342 mg
Iron	6.3 mg	Magnesium	346 mg
Phosphorus	559 mg	Potassium	2.4 g
Sodium	33 mg	Zinc	3.5 mg
Copper	810 mcg	Manganese	2.2 mg
Selenium	24 mcg	Fluoride	19 mcg
Vitamin A	15 IU	Vitamin C	8.5 mg
Thiamin	0.98 mg	Riboflavin	407 mcg
Niacin	3.8 mg	Vitamin B_6	738 mcg
Folic acid	734 mcg	Pantothenic acid	1.5 mg

- Low in calories.
- Rich in dietary fiber so acts as a bulk laxative.
- Reduces blood cholesterol levels.
- Contains zeaxanthin which prevents age related macular diseases.
- Rich in copper which prevents rheumatoid arthritis.
- Adequate source of magnesium which protects against fatigue, asthma and migraine headaches.
- Regulates the blood sugar so good for diabetics.
- Decreases the risk of atherosclerosis.
- Good source of folic acid which prevents neural tube defects in the offspring.
- Good source of potassium which controls the heart rate and blood pressure.
- Rich in iron.
- Good source of molybdenum that helps in detoxification of sulfites from the blood.

CORN

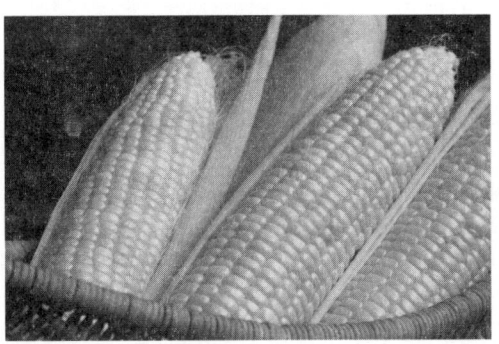

(Amount: 1 cup)			
Energy	132 calories	Carbohydrates	29 g
Proteins	5 g	Dietary fiber	3.6 g
Sugar	7.3 g	Fat	1.9 g
Calcium	3.1 mg	Iron	801 mcg
Magnesium	57 mg	Phosphorus	137 mg
Potassium	416 mg	Sodium	23 mg
Zinc	701 mcg	Copper	83 mcg
Manganese	249 mcg	Selenium	0.92 mcg
Vitamin A	145 IU	Vitamin C	10 mg
Vitamin E	108 mcg	Vitamin K	0.46 mcg
Thiamin	273 mcg	Riboflavin	89 mcg
Niacin	2.7 mg	Vitamin B_6	114 mcg
Folic acid	68 mcg	Pantothenic acid	1.1 mg

- Rich in energy.
- Rich in thiamin and niacin.
- Good source of pantothenic acid.
- Rich in vitamin B_{12} and folic acid which prevents megaloblastic anemia.
- Corn husk oil lowers plasma LDL cholesterol.
- Useful in hypertension.
- Useful in non-insulin dependent diabetes mellitus.
- Rich source of magnesium, manganese, zinc, iron, copper, selenium and phosphorus.

- Excellent source of tocopherols—an antioxidant.
- Useful in constipation and hemorrhoids.
- Prevents neural-tube birth defects.
- Prevents the cardiovascular diseases.
- Rich source of beta-carotene which is essential for maintenance of good vision and skin.
- Rich source of antioxidants which fight against the malignancy causing free radicals.
- Rich source of a phenolic compound and ferulic acid which are an anti-malignancy agent especially breast malignancy and liver malignancy.

GINGER

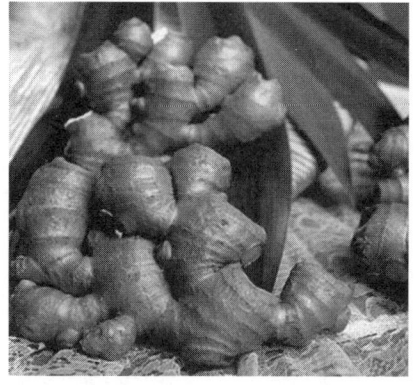

(Per 100 gm)			
Energy	80 kcal	Carbohydrates	17.77 g
Protein	1.82 g	Fat	0.75 g
Cholesterol	0 mg	Dietary fiber	2.0 g
Sodium	13 mg	Potassium	415 mg
Calcium	16 mg	Iron	0.60 mg
Magnesium	43 mg	Manganese	0.229 mg
Phosphorus	34 mg	Zinc	0.34 mg
Folic acid	11 µg	Niacin	0.750 mg
Pantothenic acid	0.203 mg	Pyridoxine	0.160 mg
Vitamin A	0 IU	Vitamin C	5 mg
Vitamin E	0.26 mg	Vitamin K	0.1 µg

- Helpful in blocking the harmful effects of prostaglandin that leads to inflammation of the blood vessels in the brain and causes migraines.
- Ginger tea has refreshing properties.
- Useful in motion sickness, migraine and also in pregnancy.
- It boosts up immune system.
- Rich in potassium, copper, magnesium and manganese.
- Decreases feeling of nausea.
- Decreases pain of rheumatoid arthritis.
- Useful in cold and flu, treating diarrhea.
- Relieving stress.
- Natural mouth freshener.
- Helpful in digestion.
- Lowers cholesterol.
- Protects against ovarian malignancy.
- Relieves menstrual cramps.

CARDAMOM /ILAICHI

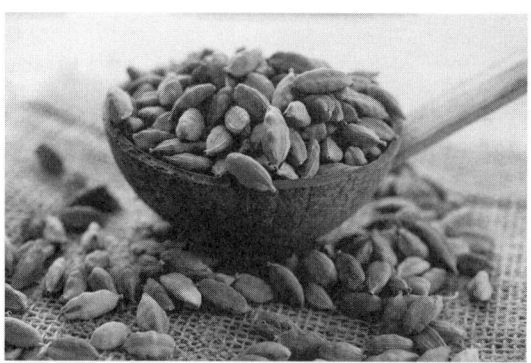

(Per 100 gm)			
Energy	311 kcal	Carbohydrates	68.47 g
Protein	10.76 g	Fat	6.7 g
Cholesterol	0 mg	Dietary fiber	28 g
Sodium	18 mg	Potassium	1119 mg

(contd.)

(*contd.*)

Calcium	383 mg	Copper	0.383 mg
Iron	13.97 mg	Magnesium	229 mg
Manganese	28 mg	Phosphorus	178 mg
Zinc	7.47 mg	Niacin	1.102 mg
Pyridoxine	0.230 mg	Riboflavin	0.182 mg
Thiamin	0.198 mg	Vitamin A	0 IU
Vitamin C	21 mg		

- It has stimulative, digestive and carminative properties.
- Enhances appetite, relieves indigestion, gas, flatulence, constipation, acidity, nausea, colic, spasms, and dysentery.
- Treats mouth ulcers, halitosis, teeth and gum infections—antibacterial action.
- Contains aromatic flavored essential volatile oil-anethole.
- Rich in pyridoxine, niacin, riboflavin, and thiamin.
- Rich in calcium, iron, copper, potassium, manganese, zinc and magnesium.
- Good source of antioxidant vitamin C and vitamin A.
- Relieves running nose.
- Seeds are chewed after a meal in India to refresh the breath.
- Used to treat menstrual cramps.
- Used as an insecticide against head-lice and mites.
- Acts as an expectorant in—sore throat, colds, coughs and respiratory allergies.
- Useful in urinary tract infection.
- It is antidote to scorpion and snake bites.
- Contains phytochemicals indole-3-carbinol and di-indolyl-methane which protects against malignancies of the breast, ovary and prostrate.
- Lowers blood pressure.

FOX NUT

(Makhana, Phool Makhana, Lotus Seeds, Gorgon Nut, Euryale Ferox)

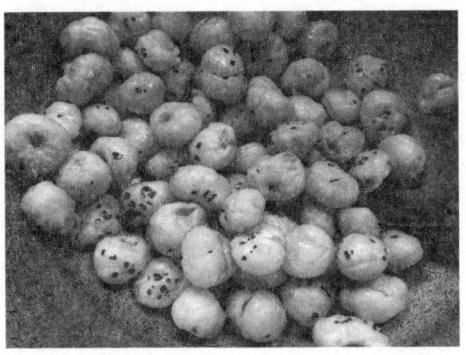

Proteins	9.7%	Carbohydrate	76%
Moisture	12.8%	Fat	0.1%
Total minerals	0.5%	Phosphorus	0.9%
Iron	1.4% mg/100 gm		

- High in fiber—relieves constipation, helpful in diarrhea and helps in improving appetite.
- Contains flavonoids—helpful in diabetes mellitus, heart diseases and malignancies.
- Powerful antioxidants and antiaging diet.
- Useful in pregnancy and postnatal weaknesses.
- Low in calories, fat and high in fiber, good food for diabetics.
- Low in saturated fats, sodium and cholesterol.
- High in magnesium, potassium and phosphorus.
- Increases quality and quantity of semen, prevents premature ejaculation, increases libido and useful in female infertility.
- Useful in frequent urination.
- Regulate the blood pressure—low in sodium and high in potassium.
- Treats insomnia, palpitations and irritability.
- Alleviates vata and pitta dosha.
- Reduces burning sensation and quenches thirst.

KHAS-KHAS (Poppy Seeds)

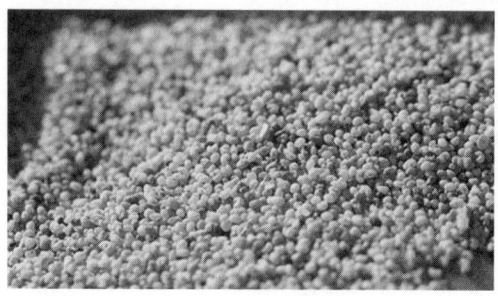

(Per 100 gm)			
Energy	525 kcal	Carbohydrates	28 g
Sugars	3 g	Dietary fiber	23 g
Fat	42 g	Saturated	5 g
Protein	18 g	Folic acid	82 µg
Vitamin E	1.8 mg	Calcium	1438 mg
Iron	10 mg	Manganese	7 mg

- Good levels of iron, copper, calcium, potassium, manganese, zinc and magnesium.
- Treats vomiting and nausea.
- Cures insomnia, asthma and cough.
- Cures under eyes dark circles.
- Useful in gout, arthritis and rheumatism.
- Contains very small quantity of opium alkaloids such as morphine, thebaine, codiene and papaverine which has beneficial effects like soothing of nervous irritability and pain killers.
- Rich in carbohydrate which increases the energy levels.
- Good source of fatty acids, rich in omega-3 fatty acids which protects heart diseases.
- Contains oleic acid which is useful in treatment of breast malignancy.
- Contains dietary fiber which helps in constipation and decrease in blood LDL cholesterol.
- Excellent source of thiamin, riboflavin, niacin, pantothenic acid, pyridoxine and folic acid.
- Not recommended for pregnant women since it causes nausea.

TURMERIC

Indian Saffron

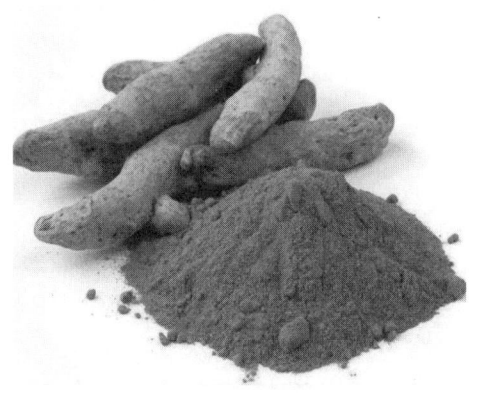

	(Per 100 gm)		
Energy	354 kcal	Carbohydrates	64.9 g
Protein	7.83 g	Fat	9.88 g
Cholesterol	0 mg	Dietary fiber	21 g
Sodium	38 mg	Potassium	2525 mg
Calcium	183 mg	Copper	603 µg
Iron	41.42 mg	Magnesium	193 mg
Manganese	7.83 mg	Phosphorus	268 mg
Zinc	4.35 mg	Folic acid	39 µg
Niacin	5.140 mg	Pyridoxine	1.80 mg
Riboflavin	0.233 mg	Vitamin A	0 IU
Vitamin C	25.9 mg	Vitamin E	3.10 mg
Vitamin K	13.4 µg		

- Rich in pyridoxine, choline, niacin, and riboflavin which are essential for good health.
- Useful in treatment of homocystinuria, sideroblastic anemia and radiation sickness.
- Have anti-inflammatory, carminative, anti-flatulent and anti-microbial properties.
- Contains curcumin, a poly-phenolic compound helpful against multiple myeloma, pancreatic malignancy, and colon malignancy.

- Prevents Alzheimer's disease.
- Useful in dental infections, sinus conditions, menstrual difficulties, parasites, jaundice, diarrhea, and colic.
- Lowers blood sugar.
- Used for epilepsy.
- Rich in calcium, iron, potassium, manganese, copper, zinc and magnesium.
- Good levels of vitamin C—a powerful natural anti-oxidant.
- A paste applied on skin improves complexion, cures rashes, boils, infections, eczema, acne and wound.
- Has anti-tumor, antioxidant, anti-arthritic, anti-amyloid, anti-ischemic, and anti-inflammatory properties.
- Rich in dietary fiber, which controls "bad cholesterol".

CORIANDER

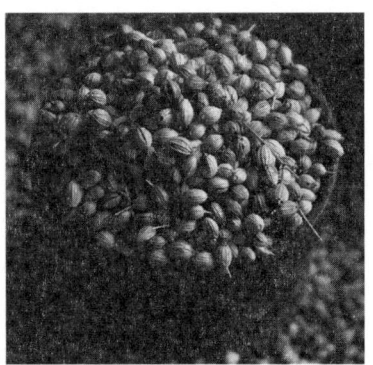

(Per 100 gm)			
Energy	298 kcal	Carbohydrates	54.99 g
Protein	12.37 g	Fat	17.77 g
Cholesterol	0 mg	Dietary fiber	41.9 g
Sodium	35 mg	Potassium	1267 mg
Calcium	709 mg	Copper	0.975 mg
Iron	16.32 mg	Magnesium	330 mg
Manganese	1.900 mg	Phosphorus	409 mg
Zinc	4.70 mg	Folic acid	1 µg
Niacin	2.130 mg	Riboflavin	0.290 mg
Thiamin	0.239 mg	Vitamin A	0 IU
Vitamin C	21 mg		

- A Chinese parsley
- Has antioxidant properties.
- Good source of dietary fiber which decreases LDL cholesterol, also reduces the risk of heart attack.
- Rich in iron, copper, calcium, potassium, manganese, magnesium and zinc.
- Relieves tension, migraine nervous weakness, arthritic pains, muscle spasms
- Folk medicine for anxiety and insomnia and indigestion.
- Rich aroma which is excellent appetizer.
- High levels of vitamin C.
- Rich in thiamine, niacin and riboflavin.
- Rich in vitamin K.
- Useful in the treatment of Alzheimer's disease.
- Cures heavy menstrual flow.
- Maintains low blood sugar by stimulating the secretion of insulin.

DRUMSTICKS

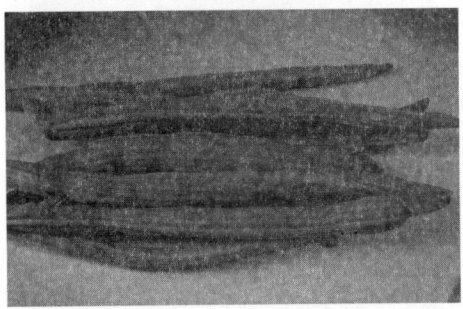

(Per 100 gm)			
Energy	26 kcal	Carbohydrates	3.7 g
Dietary fiber	4.8 g	Fat	0.4 g
Protein	9.8 g	Water	86.9 g
Vitamin A	7564 IU	Vitamin C	120 mg
Calcium	30 mg	Iron	5.3 mg
Phosphorus	110 mg	Potassium	134 mg

- Fresh pods and seeds are a good source of oleic acid, a health-benefiting monounsaturated fat.
- Rich in vitamin A which maintains skin integrity, vision, and immunity.
- Good in folic acid, vitamin B$_6$, thiamin, riboflavin, pantothenic acid and niacin.
- Rich in calcium, iron, copper, manganese, zinc, selenium, and magnesium.
- Good in vitamin C which gives immunity against infectious agents and harmful oxygen-free radicals.

PEAS

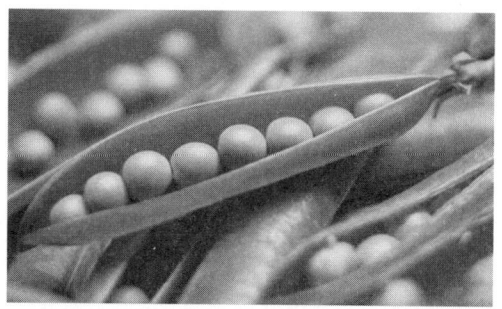

(Per 100 gm)			
Energy	81 kcal	Carbohydrates	14.45 g
Dietary fiber	5.1 g	Fat	0.4 g
Protein	5.42 g	Calcium	25 mg
Iron	1.47 mg	Magnesium	33 mg
Phosphorus	108 mg	Potassium	244 mg
Zinc	1.24 mg	Vitamin A	38 µg
Vitamin B$_3$	2.09 mg	Vitamin B$_6$	0.169 mg
Vitamin B$_9$	65 µg	Vitamin C	40 mg
Vitamin E	0.13 mg	Vitamin K	24.8 µg

- Boosts up immunity.
- Useful in prevention of wrinkles, Alzheimer's disese, arthritis, bronchitis and osteoporosis.
- Makes bones healthy.

- Lowers VLDL cholesterol.
- Regulates blood sugar.
- Prevents stomach malignancy.
- Rich in nitrogen.
- Prevents heart diseases and constipation.

PUMPKIN

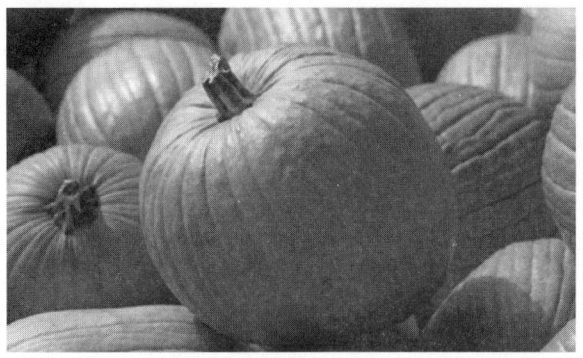

(Per 100 gm)			
Energy	26 kcal	Carbohydrates	6.5 g
Dietary fiber	0.5 g	Fat	0.1 g
Protein	1 g	Calcium	21 mg
Iron	0.8 mg	Magnesium	12 mg
Phosphorus	44 mg	Potassium	340 mg
Zinc	0.32 mg	Vitamin A	426 µg
Vitamin B_3	0.6 mg	Vitamin B_5	0.298 mg
Vitamin B_9	16 µg	Vitamin C	9 mg
Vitamin E	0.44 mg	Vitamin K	1.1 µg

- Easily absorbable and good quality of proteins
- Natural treatment for tapeworms and other parasites.
- Lowers LDL (bad cholesterol).
- Helpful in difficult urination in benign enlargement of prostate.
- Prevents calcium oxalate kidney stones formation.
- Reduces inflammation of arthritis.

PARSLEY ROOT

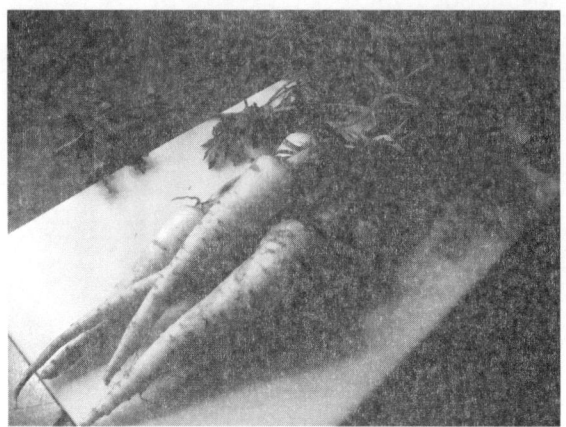

- Rich in vitamins A, C and K.
- Rich in copper, iron and iodine.
- Used in greek medicine to treat flatulence, indigestion, spasms and menstrual disorders.
- Useful for treating chronic liver and gallbladder diseases.
- High in sodium, folic acid, potassium, calcium, phosphorus, protein and fiber.
- Strong antioxidant.

CASAVA

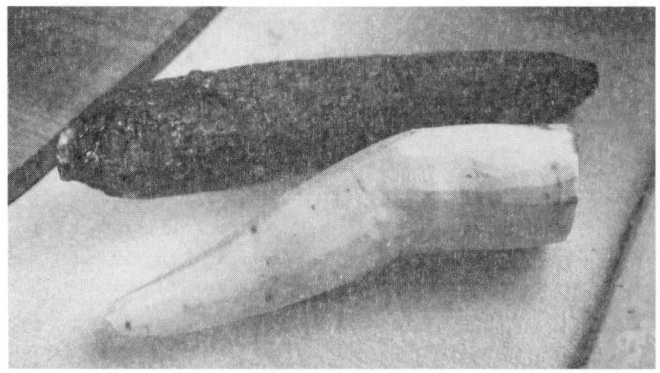

(Per 100 gm)			
Energy	160 kcal	Carbohydrates	38.06 g
Protein	1.36 g	Fat	0.28 g
Cholesterol	0 mg	Dietary fiber	1.8 g
Sodium	14 mg	Potassium	271 mg
Calcium	16 mg	Iron	0.27 mg
Magnesium	21 mg	Manganese	0.383 mg
Phosphorus	27 µg	Zinc	0.34 mg
Folic acid	27 µg	Niacin	0.854 mg
Pyridoxine	0.088 mg	Riboflavin	0.048 mg
Thiamin	0.087 mg	Vitamin A	13 IU
Vitamin C	20.6 mg	Vitamin E	0.19 mg
Vitamin K	1.9 µg		

- Very low in fats and protein.
- Free from gluten so useful in celiac disease.
- Moderate source of folic acid, thiamin, pyridoxine, riboflavin and pantothenic acid.
- Rich in zinc, magnesium, copper, iron, and manganese.

SWEET POTATO ROOT

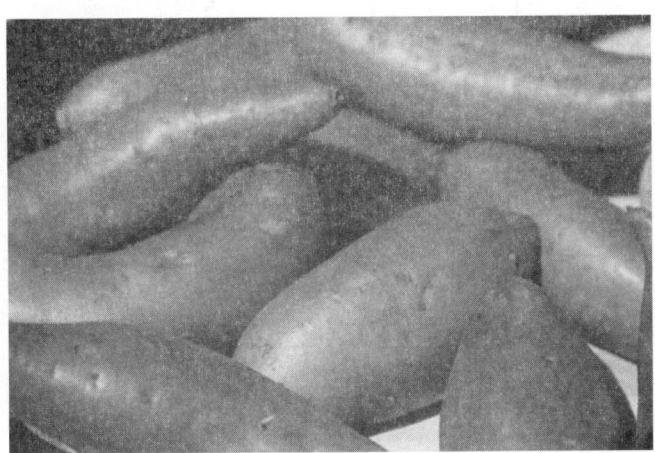

(Per 100 gm)			
Energy	86 kcal	Carbohydrates	20.1 g
Starch	12.7 g	Sugars	4.2 g
Dietary fibre	3 g	Fat	0.1 g
Protein	1.6 g	Calcium	30 mg
Iron	0.61 mg	Magnesium	25 mg
Manganese	0.258 mg	Phosphorus	47 mg
Potassium	337 mg	Sodium	55 mg
Zinc	0.3 mg	Vitamin A	709 µg
Beta-carotene	8509 µg	Thiamine	0.078 mg
Riboflavin	0.061 mg	Niacin	0.557 mg
Pantothenic acid	0.8 mg	Vitamin B_6	0.209 mg
Folic acid	11 µg	Vitamin C	2.4 mg
Vitamin E	0.26 mg		

- Starchy and sweet-tasting.
- Highest in nutritional value.
- Rich in carbohydrates, dietary fiber, beta-carotene and vitamin C, vitamin B_6.
- Rich in minerals such as iron, calcium, magnesium, manganese, and potassium.
- Contains no saturated fats or cholesterol.
- Rich in pantothenic acid, pyridoxine, thiamin, niacin, riboflavin.

SWEET POTATO LEAVES

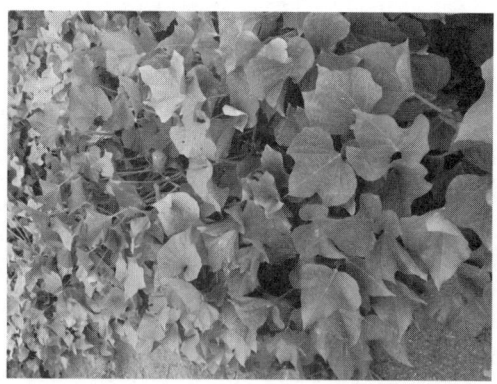

(Per 100 gm)			
Energy	42 kcal	Carbohydrates	8.82 g
Dietary fiber	5.3 g	Fat	0.51 g
Protein	2.49 g	Calcium	78 mg
Iron	0.97 mg	Magnesium	70 mg
Phosphorus	81 mg	Potassium	508 mg
Vitamin A	189 µg	Beta-carotene	2217 µg
Lutein and zeaxanthin	14720 µg	Thiamine	0.156 mg
Riboflavin	0.345 mg	Niacin	1.13 mg
Pantothenic acid	0.225 mg	Vitamin B_6	0.19 mg
Vitamin C	11 mg	Vitamin K	302.2 µg

- Leaves are more nutritious than the tuber itself.
- Rich in iron, vitamin C, folic acid, vitamin K, and potassium.

YAM

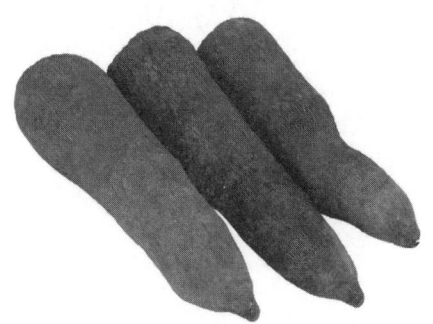

(Per 100 gm)			
Energy	118 kcal	Carbohydrates	27.9 g
Sugars	0.5 g	Dietary fiber	4.1 g
Fat	0.17 g	Protein	1.5 g
Calcium	17 mg	Iron	0.54 mg
Magnesium	21 mg	Manganese	0.397 mg
Phosphorus	55 mg	Potassium	816 mg
Zinc	0.24 mg	Vitamin A	7 µg
Thiamine	0.112 mg	Riboflavin	0.032 mg
Niacin	0.552 mg	Pantothenic acid	0.314 mg
Vitamin B_6	0.293 mg	Folic acid	23 µg
Vitamin C	17.1 mg	Vitamin E	0.35 mg
Vitamin K	2.3 µg		

- Edible tubers.
- Low in protein content so in areas of Africa have a high incidence of kwashiorkor.
- Lower glycemic index.
- Contains thiocyanate which protects against sickle cell anemia.
- Rich in phenylalanine and threonine.
- Low nutrient density.
- High in vitamins C and B_6, potassium, manganese and dietary fiber.
- Low in saturated fat and sodium.
- Protects against osteoporosis and heart disease.

PLANTAIN (Cooking Bananas)

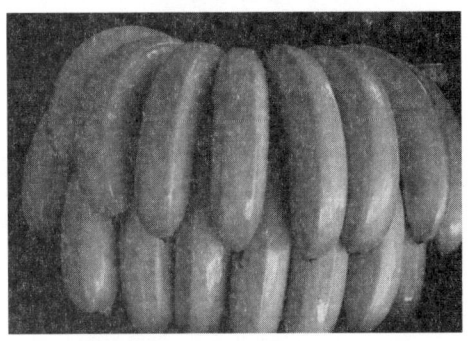

(Per 100 gm)			
Energy	120 kcal	Carbohydrates	31.89 g
Sugars	15 g	Dietary fiber	2.3 g
Fat	0.37 g	Calcium	3 mg
Iron	0.6 mg	Magnesium	37 mg
Phosphorus	34 mg	Potassium	499 mg
Sodium	4 mg	Zinc	0.14 mg
Protein	1.3 g	Vitamin A	56 µg
Beta-carotene	457 µg	Thiamine	0.052 mg
Riboflavin	0.054 mg	Niacin	0.686 mg
Pantothenic acid	0.26 mg	Vitamin B_6	0.299 mg
Folic acid	22 µg	Choline	13.5 mg
Vitamin C	18.4 mg	Vitamin E	0.14 mg
Vitamin K	0.7 µg		

- Rich in carbohydrate and starch.
- Low in fat
- Ideal food for geriatric patients.
- Ideal food for gastric ulcer, coeliac disease and colitis.
- Contains very little beta-carotene.

TARO

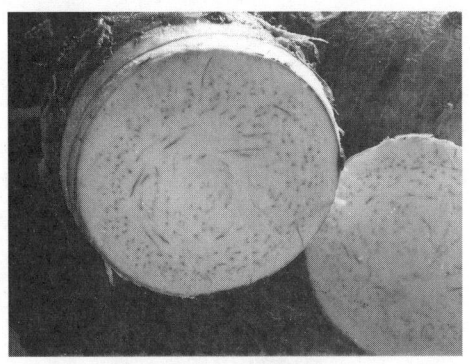

(Per 100 gm)			
Energy	142 kcal	Carbohydrates	34.6 g
Sugars	0.49 g	Dietary fiber	5.1 g
Fat	0.11 g	Protein	0.52 g
Calcium	18 mg	Iron	0.72 mg
Magnesium	30 mg	Manganese	0.449 mg
Phosphorus	76 mg	Potassium	484 mg
Zinc	0.27 mg	Thiamine	0.107 mg
Riboflavin	0.028 mg	Niacin	0.51 mg
Pantothenic acid	0.336 mg	Vitamin B_6	0.331 mg
Folic acid	19 µg	Vitamin C	5 mg
Vitamin E	2.93 mg		

- Root vegetable.
- Rich in dietary fiber.
- Rich in protein.
- Rich in calcium, vitamin C, vitamin E and B vitamins, as well as magnesium, manganese and copper.

- Caution—lead to kidney stones and gout.
- Have low glycemic index which prevents diabetes.
- Excellent source of potassium.

TARO LEAVES

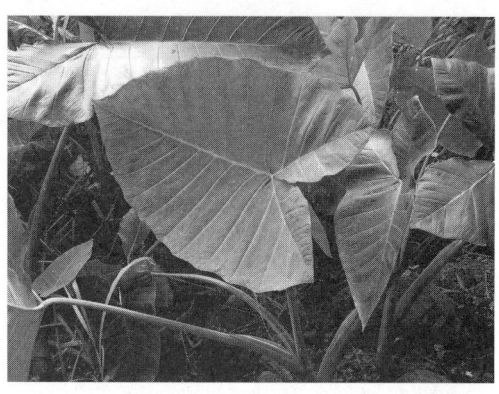

(Per 100 gm)			
Energy	42 kcal	Carbohydrates	6.7 g
Sugars	3 g	Dietary fiber	3.7 g
Fat	0.74 g	Protein	5 g
Calcium	107 mg	Iron	2.25 mg
Magnesium	45 mg	Manganese	0.714 mg
Phosphorus	60 mg	Potassium	648 mg
Zinc	0.41 mg	Vitamin A	241 µg
Thiamine	0.209 mg	Riboflavin	0.456 mg
Niacin	1.513 mg	Vitamin B_6	0.146 mg
Folic acid	126 µg	Vitamin C	52 mg
Vitamin E	2.02 mg	Vitamin K	108.6 µg

- Controls blood pressure and blood sugar, protects from cardiovascular disease and malignancy.
- Rich in calcium, iron, magnesium, manganese, phosphorous, sodium, zinc and selenium.
- Rich in omega-3 and omega-6 fatty acids.
- Contains vitamins A, C, E, K, thiamin, niacin, riboflavin, B_6, folic acid B_{12} and pantothenic acid and choline.

SHALLOT (Allium Cepa)

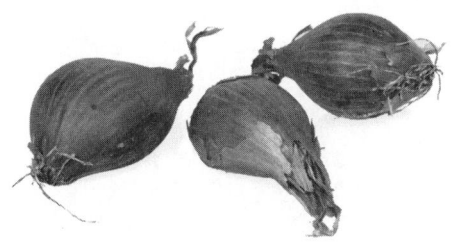

	(Per 100 gm)		
Energy	72 kcal	Carbohydrates	16.8 g
Sugars	7.87 g	Dietary fiber	3.2 g
Fat	0.1 g	Protein	2.5 g
Calcium	37 mg	Iron	1.2 mg
Thiamine	0.06 mg	Riboflavin	0.02 mg
Niacin	0.2 mg	Pantothenic acid	0.29 mg
Vitamin B_6	0.345 mg	Folic acid	34 µg
Vitamin C	8 mg		

- Magnesium—21 mg
- Manganese—0.292 mg
- Phosphorus—60 mg
- Potassium—334 mg
- Zinc—0.4 mg

RAW ONIONS

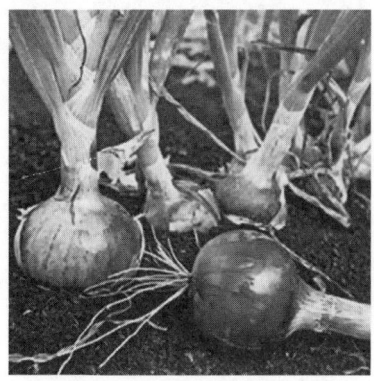

(Per 100 gm)			
Energy	40 kcal	Carbohydrates	9.34 g
Sugars	4.24 g	Dietary fiber	1.7 g
Fat	0.1 g	Protein	1.1 g
Calcium	23 mg	Iron	0.21 mg
Magnesium	10 mg	Manganese	0.129 mg
Phosphorus	29 mg	Potassium	146 mg
Zinc	0.17 mg	Fluoride	1.1 µg
Thiamine	0.046 mg	Riboflavin	0.027 mg
Niacin	0.116 mg	Pantothenic acid	0.123 mg
Vitamin B_6	0.12 mg	Folic acid	19 µg
Vitamin C	7.4 mg		

- Contains phenolic and flavonoids which have anti-inflammatory, anti-cholesterol, antimalignancy and antioxidant properties.

TOMATILLO OR TOMATE

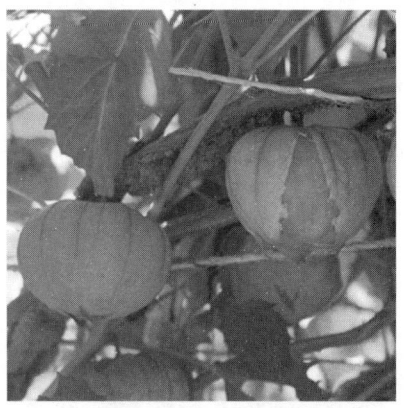

Energy	32 kcal	Carbohydrates	5.84 g
Protein	0.96 g	Fat	1.02 g
Cholesterol	0 mg	Dietary fiber	1.9 g
Sodium	1 mg	Potassium	268 mg
Calcium	7 mg	Copper	0.079 mg
Iron	0.62 mg	Magnesium	20 mg
Manganese	0.153 mg	Phosphorus	39 mg
Selenium	0.5 µg	Zinc	0.22 mg

(contd.)

Folic acid	7 µg	Niacin	1.850 mg
Pyridoxine	0.056 mg	Thiamin	0.044 mg
Vitamin A	114 IU	Vitamin C	11.7 mg
Vitamin E	0.38 mg	Vitamin K	10.1 µg

- Low in calories.
- Does not contain lycopene.
- Have anti-bacterial and anti-malignancy properties.
- Less in vitamins A, C, and E.
- Rich in sodium, copper, iron, phosphorous and manganese.

PUMPKIN SEEDS

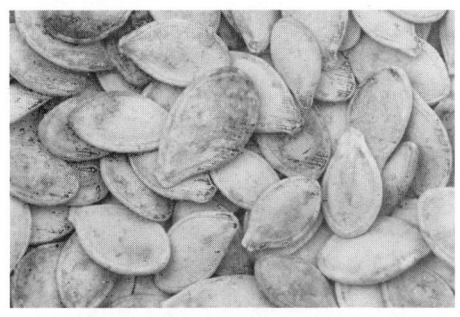

Energy	559 kcal	Carbohydrates	10.71 g
Protein	30.23 g	Fat	49.05 g
Cholesterol	0 mg	Dietary fiber	6 g
Sodium	7 mg	Potassium	809 mg
Calcium	46 mg	Copper	1.343 mg
Iron	8.82 mg	Magnesium	592 mg
Manganese	4.543 mg	Phosphorus	1233 mg
Selenium	9.4 µg	Zinc	7.81 mg
Folic acid	58 µg	Niacin	4.987 mg
Pantothenic acid	0.750 mg	Pyridoxine	0.143 mg
Riboflavin	0.153 mg	Thiamin	0.273 mg
Vitamin A	16 IU	Vitamin C	1.9 µg
Vitamin E	35.10 mg		

- High in calories.
- Rich in mono-unsaturated fatty acids that helps lower bad cholesterol and increases good cholesterol.

- Rich in copper, manganese, potassium, calcium, iron, magnesium, zinc and selenium.
- Prevents prostate and ovarian malignancies also diabetic nephropathy.
- Rich in protein-amino acid like tryptophan and glutamate.
- Rich in vitamin E, thiamin, riboflavin, niacin, pantothenic acid, vitamin B_6 and folic acid.

PEPPERMINT

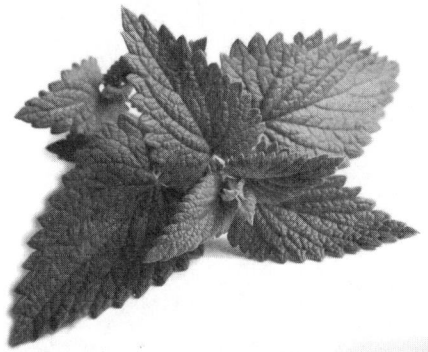

Energy	70 kcal	Carbohydrates	14.79 g
Protein	3.75 g	Fat	0.94 g
Cholesterol	0 mg	Dietary fiber	8 g
Sodium	31 mg	Potassium	569 mg
Calcium	243 mg	Copper	329 µg
Iron	5.08 mg	Magnesium	80 mg
Manganese	1.176 mg	Zinc	1.11 mg
Folic acid	114 µg	Niacin	1.706 mg
Pantothenic acid	0.338 mg	Pyridoxine	0.129 mg
Riboflavin	0.266 mg	Thiamin	0.082 mg
Vitamin A	4248 IU	Vitamin C	31.8 mg

- Cholesterol free.
- Rich in essential oils, vitamins and dietary fiber which helps to control blood cholesterol and blood pressure.
- Contains many essential volatile oils like menthol, menthone, menthol acetate which have natural cooling sensation.

- Rich in potassium, calcium, iron, manganese and magnesium.
- Rich in vitamin A, beta carotene, vitamin C, vitamin E, folic acid, riboflavin and pyridoxine and vitamin K.
- Menthol is analgesic and local anesthetic.
- It relaxes intestinal wall and sphincter smooth muscles through blocking calcium channel at cell receptor levels.
- Have anti-spasmodic action, so used in management of irritable bowel syndrome.

RAW LEEKS (A. Ampeloprasum var. porrum)

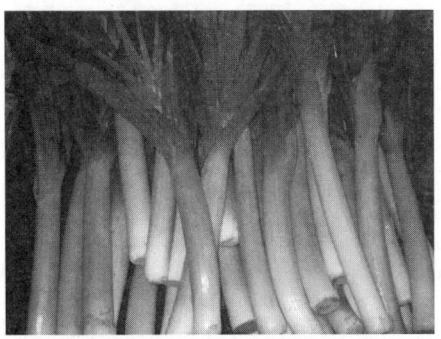

(Per 100 gm)			
Energy	61 kcal	Carbohydrates	14.15 g
Sugars	3.9 g	Dietary fiber	1.8 g
Fat	0.3 g	Protein	1.5 g
Calcium	59 mg	Iron	2.1 mg
Magnesium	28 mg	Manganese	0.481 mg
Phosphorus	35 mg	Potassium	180 mg
Vitamin A	83 µg	Thiamine	0.06 mg
Riboflavin	0.03 mg	Niacin	0.4 mg
Pantothenic acid	0.14 mg	Vitamin B$_6$	0.233 mg
Folic acid	64 µg	Vitamin C	12 mg
Vitamin E	0.92 mg	Vitamin K	47 µg

- Low in calories.
- Good amount of soluble and insoluble fiber.
- Reduces cholesterol production by inhibiting the HMG-CoA reductase enzyme.

- Rich in vitamins A, C, K, and E.
- Small amount of potassium, iron, calcium, magnesium, manganese, zinc, and selenium.
- Have anti-bacterial, anti-viral and anti-fungal activities.
- Decreases risk of coronary artery disease, peripheral vascular diseases and stroke.
- Rich in pyridoxine, folic acid, niacin, riboflavin, and thiamin and thus prevents neural tube defects in the newborn babies.

GREEN BEANS

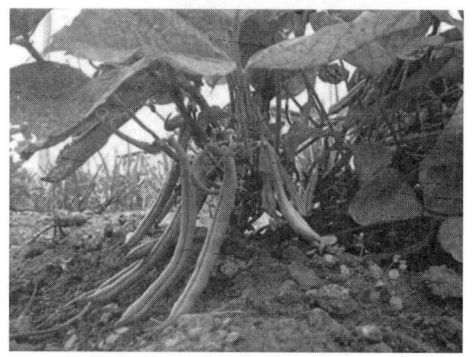

Energy	31 kcal	Carbohydrates	7.13 g
Protein	1.82 g	Fat	0.34 g
Cholesterol	0 mg	Dietary fiber	3.4 g
Sodium	6 mg	Potassium	209 mg
Calcium	37 mg	Iron	1.04 mg
Magnesium	25 mg	Manganese	0.214 mg
Phosphorus	38 mg	Zinc	0.24 mg
Folic acid	37 µg	Niacin	0.752 mg
Pantothenic acid	0.094 mg	Pyridoxine	0.074 mg
Riboflavin	0.105 mg	Thiamin	0.084 mg
Vitamin A	690 IU	Vitamin C	16.3 mg
Vitamin K	14.4 µg		

- Low in calories.
- No saturated fat.
- Also rich in iron, calcium, magnesium, manganese, and potassium.

- Rich in dietary fiber which reduces blood cholesterol.
- Rich in vitamin A, lutein, zeaxanthin and β-carotene, folic acid, vitamin B_6, thiamin and vitamin C.

POINTED GOURD–PARWAL

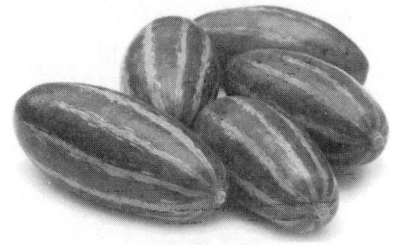

- Rich in vitamins A, B_1, B_2, and C.
- Rich in calcium, phosphorous, iron, copper and potassium.
- As per ayurveda useful for kapha.
- Stimulates digestion.

RIDGE GOURD

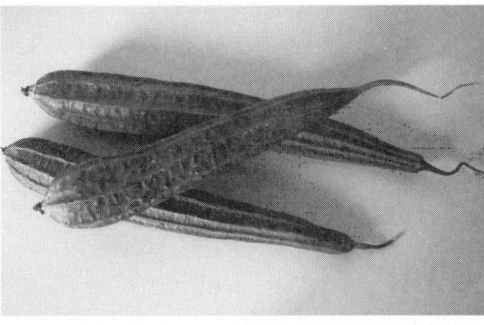

- Low in fat and calories.
- Low in saturated fat and cholesterol.
- Helps to lower blood and urine sugar levels without altering blood insulin levels.
- Relieves constipation and cures piles.
- High in dietary fiber.
- Very high water content.

- Natural remedy for jaundice.
- Protects liver from alcohol intoxication.

CARDOON

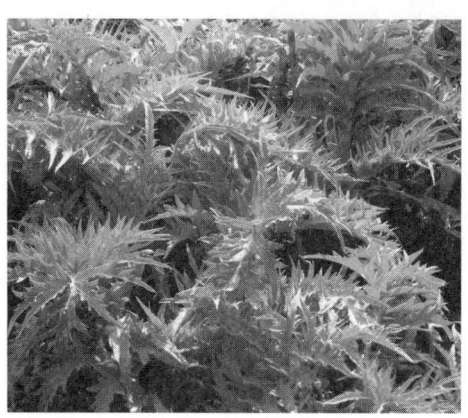

Energy	17 kcal	Carbohydrates	4.07 g
Protein	0.70 g	Fat	0.10 g
Cholesterol	0 mg	Dietary fiber	1.6 g
Sodium	170 mg	Potassium	400 mg
Calcium	70 mg	Copper	0.231 mg
Iron	0.70 mg	Magnesium	42 mg
Manganese	0.256 mg	Phosphorus	23 mg
Selenium	0.2 µg	Zinc	0.17 mg
Folic acid	68 µg	Niacin	0.300 mg
Pantothenic acid	0.338 mg	Pyridoxine	0.116 mg
Riboflavin	0.030 mg	Thiamin	0.020 mg
Vitamin C	2 mg	Vitamin A	0 IU

- Very low calorie.
- Reduces cholesterol.
- Rich in folic acid, niacin, vitamin B_6, thiamin, and pantothenic acid.
- Rich source of copper, calcium, potassium, iron, manganese, and phosphorus.

- Contains phytonutrients as luteolin, silymarin, caffeic, ferulic and dicaffeoyl-quinic acids, which protect cellular proteins and DNA from oxidative damage caused by free radicals.

SWISS CHARD

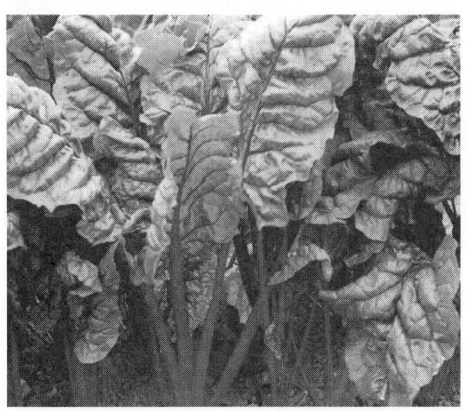

Carbohydrates	3.74 g	Protein	3.27 g
Fat	0.20 g	Cholesterol	0 mg
Dietary fiber	1.6 g	Sodium	213 mg
Potassium	379 mg	Calcium	51 mg
Copper	0.179 mg	Iron	1.80 mg
Magnesium	81 mg	Manganese	0.366 mg
Phosphorus	46 mg	Selenium	0.9 µg
Zinc	0.39 mg	Folic acid	14 µg
Niacin	0.400 mg	Pantothenic acid	0.172 mg
Pyridoxine	0.99 mg	Riboflavin	0.090 mg
Thiamin	0.040 mg	Vitamin A	6116 IU
Vitamin C	30 mg	Vitamin E	1.89 mg
Vitamin K	830 µg		

- Low in calories and fats.
- Rich source of copper, calcium, sodium, potassium, iron, manganese and phosphorus.
- Rich in vitamin C, vitamin K, omega-3 fatty acids; vitamin A, and flavonoids antioxidants like β-carotene.

- Rich in folic acid, niacin, vitamin B_6, thiamin and pantothenic acid.

COLLARD GREENS

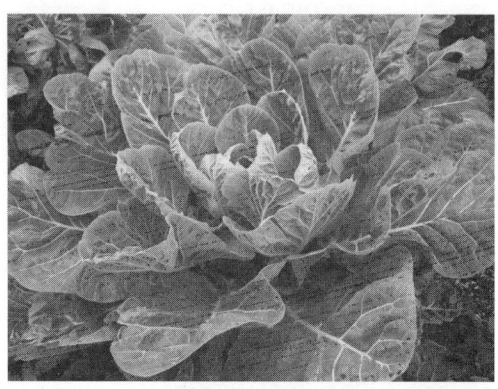

(Per 100 gm)			
Energy	30 kcal	Carbohydrates	5.69 g
Protein	2.45 g	Fat	0.42 g
Cholesterol	0 mg	Dietary fiber	3.60 g
Sodium	20 mg	Potassium	169 mg
Calcium	145 mg	Copper	0.039 mg
Iron	0.19 mg	Magnesium	9 mg
Manganese	0.276 mg	Selenium	1.3 µg
Zinc	0.13 mg	Folic acid	166 µg
Niacin	0.742 mg	Pantothenic acid	0.267 mg
Pyridoxine	0.165 mg	Riboflavin	0.130 mg
Thiamin	0.054 mg	Vitamin A	6668 IU
Vitamin C	35.3 mg	Vitamin E	2.26 mg
Vitamin K	510.8 µg		

- Low in calories.
- Cholesterol free.
- Rich in folic acid, vitamin C, vitamin A, vitamin K, niacin, pantothenic acid, pyridoxine and riboflavin.
- Good in iron, calcium, copper, manganese, selenium and zinc.

- Rich in soluble and insoluble dietary fiber that helps control LDL cholesterol levels and gives protection against hemorrhoids, constipation as well as colon malignancy.
- Rich in phyto-nutrients that have potent anti-malignancy action against prostate, breast, cervical, colon, ovarian cancer.

DANDELION

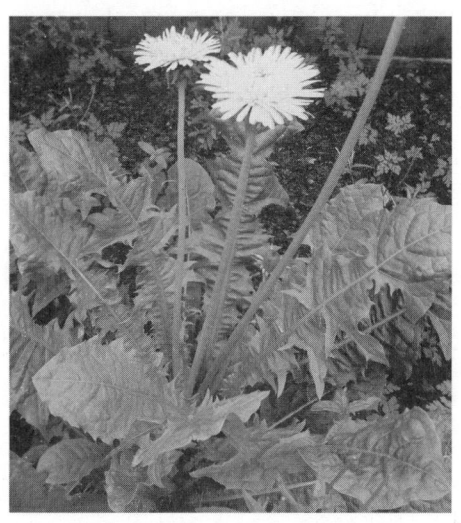

(Per 100 gm)			
Energy	45 kcal	Carbohydrates	9.20 g
Protein	2.70 g	Fat	0.70 g
Cholesterol	0 mg	Dietary fiber	3.50 g
Sodium	76 mg	Potassium	397 mg
Calcium	187 mg	Iron	3.10 mg
Magnesium	36 mg	Manganese	0.342 mg
Phosphorus	66 mg	Selenium	0.5 mg
Zinc	0.41 mg	Folic acid	27 µg
Niacin	0.806 mg	Pantothenic acid	0.084 mg
Pyridoxine	0.251 mg	Riboflavin	0.260 mg
Thiamin	0.190 mg	Vitamin A	10161 IU
Vitamin C	35 mg	Vitamin E	3.44 mg
Vitamin K	778.4 µg		

- Low in calories.
- Good source of dietary fiber.
- Rich in folic acid, riboflavin, pyridoxine, niacin, vitamin E and vitamin C.
- Richest herbal sources of vitamin K.
- Rich in vitamin A, carotene-β, carotene-α, lutein, crypto-xanthin and zeaxanthin.
- Rich in potassium, calcium, manganese, iron and magnesium.

DILL WEED

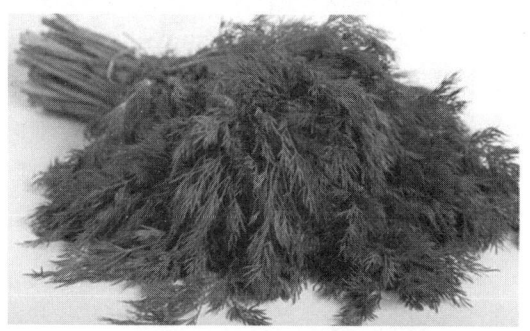

Energy	43 kcal	Carbohydrates	7 g
Protein	3.46 g	Fat	1.12 g
Cholesterol	0 mg	Dietary fiber	2.10 g
Sodium	61 mg	Potassium	738 mg
Calcium	208 mg	Copper	0.146 mg
Iron	6.59 mg	Magnesium	55 mg
Manganese	1.264 mg	Phosphorus	66 mg
Zinc	0.91 mg	Folic acid	150 µg
Niacin	1.570 mg	Pantothenic acid	0.397 mg
Pyridoxine	0.185 mg	Riboflavin	0.296 mg
Thiamin	0.058 mg	Vitamin A	7718 IU
Vitamin C	85 mg		

- Cholesterol free.
- Low in calories.
- Contains essential volatile oils such as d-carvone, dillapiol, DHC, eugenol, limonene, terpinene and myristicin.

- Acts as local anesthetic, anti-spasmodic, carminative, digestive, disinfectant, galactagogue and antiseptic.
- Rich in copper, potassium, calcium, manganese, iron, and magnesium.
- Reduces blood sugar levels in diabetics.
- Rich in folic acid, riboflavin, niacin, vitamin A, β-carotene, vitamin C.

ENDIVE

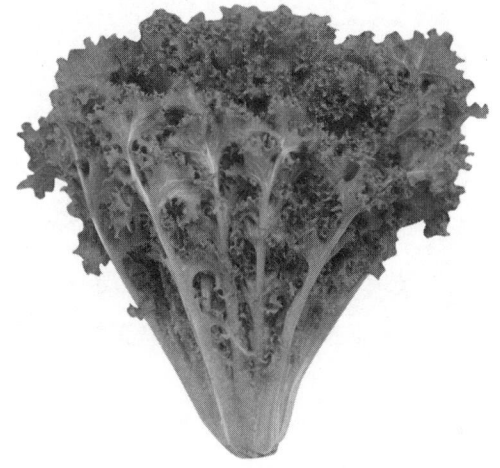

Energy	17 kcal	Carbohydrates	3.35 g
Protein	1.25 g	Fat	0.20 g
Cholesterol	0 mg	Dietary fiber	3.10 g
Sodium	22 mg	Potassium	314 mg
Calcium	52 mg	Copper	0.099 mg
Iron	0.83 mg	Magnesium	15 mg
Manganese	0.420 mg	Phosphorus	28 mg
Selenium	0.2 mcg	Zinc	0.79 mg
Folic acid	142 µg	Niacin	0.400 mg
Pantothenic acid	0.900 mg	Pyridoxine	0.020 mg
Riboflavin	0.075 mg	Thiamin	0.080 mg
Vitamin A	2167 IU	Vitamin C	6.5 mg
Vitamin E	0.44 mg	Vitamin K	231 µg

- Low calorie leafy vegetable.
- Rich in vitamin A and β-carotene, folic acid, pantothenic acid, pyridoxine thiamin, niacin.
- Rich in manganese, copper, iron, and potassium.
- High inulin and fiber content in escarole help reduce glucose and LDL cholesterol levels in diabetes and obese patients.

FENNEL BULB (Sweet Fennel)

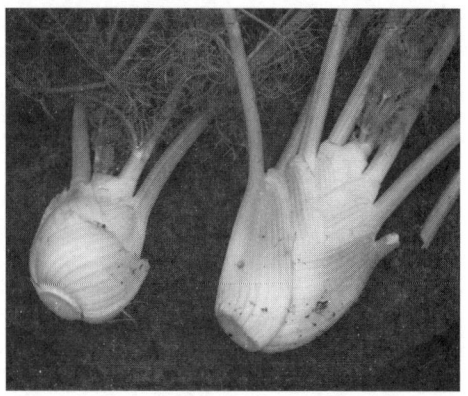

(Per 100 gm)			
Energy	31 kcal	Carbohydrates	7.29 g
Protein	1.24 g	Fat	0.20 g
Cholesterol	0 mg	Dietary fiber	3.1 g
Sodium	52 mg	Potassium	414 m
Calcium	49 mg	Copper	0.066 mg
Iron	0.73 mg	Magnesium	17 mg
Manganese	0.191 mg	Phosphorus	50 mg
Selenium	0.7 µg	Zinc	0.20 mg
Folic acid	27 µg	Niacin	0.640 mg
Pantothenic acid	0.232 mg	Pyridoxine	0.047 mg
Riboflavin	0.032 mg	Thiamin	0.010 mg
Vitamin A	134 IU	Vitamin C	12 mg

- Low calorie and fat.
- Cholesterol free.
- Rich in potassium, zinc, and selenium.

- High concentration of aromatic essential oils like anethole, estragole, and fenchone which have anti-fungal and anti-bacterial properties.
- Moderate amount of pantothenic acid, pyridoxine folic acid, niacin, riboflavin, thiamin and vitamin C.

BITTER GOURD

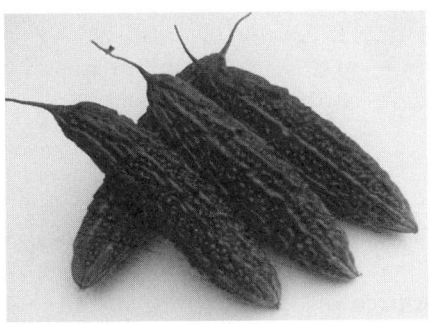

- Low in calories.
- Contains phyto-nutrient like polypeptide-P which is plant insulin lowers blood sugar levels.
- Effective for treating HIV infection.
- Rich in folic acid, vitamins C, A, β-carotene, α-carotene, lutein, and zeaxanthin.
- Good source of niacin, pantothenic acid, pyridoxine, iron, zinc, potassium, manganese and magnesium.

JICAMA (Yam Bean)

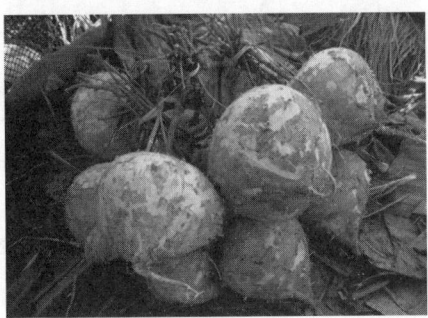

(Per 100 gm)			
Energy	38 kcal	Carbohydrates	8.82 g
Protein	0.72 g	Fat	0.19 g
Cholesterol	0 mg	Dietary fiber	4.9 g
Sodium	4 mg	Potassium	150 mg
Calcium	12 mg	Copper	0.048 mg
Iron	0.60 mg	Magnesium	12 mg
Manganese	0.60 mg	Zinc	0.16 mg
Folic acid	12 µg	Niacin	0.200 mg
Pantothenic acid	0.135 mg	Pyridoxine	0.042 mg
Riboflavin	0.029 mg	Thiamin	0.020 mg
Vitamin A	21 IU	Vitamin C	20.2 mg
Vitamin E	0.46 mg	Vitamin K	0.3 µg

- Low in calories.
- Contains finest source dietary fiber.
- Excellent source of oligofructose inulin, a soluble dietary fiber.
- Rich in magnesium, copper, iron and manganese.
- Ideal sweet snack for diabetics.
- Rich in vitamin C.
- Small amount of folic acid, riboflavin, pyridoxine, pantothenic acid and thiamin.

KOHLRABI OR KNOL-KHOL OR GERMAN TURNIP

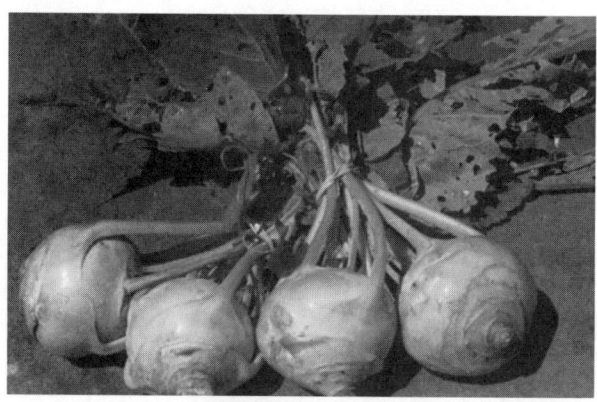

(Per 100 gm)			
Energy	27 kcal	Carbohydrates	6.20 g
Protein	1.70 g	Fat	0.10 g
Cholesterol	0 mg	Dietary fiber	3.6 g
Sodium	20 mg	Potassium	350 mg
Calcium	24 mg	Copper	0.129 mg
Iron	0.40 mg	Magnesium	19 mg
Manganese	0.139 mg	Phosphorus	46 mg
Selenium	0.7 µg	Zinc	0.03 mg
Folic acid	16 µg	Niacin	0.400 mg
Pantothenic acid	0.165 mg	Pyridoxine	0.150 mg
Riboflavin	0.020 mg	Thiamin	0.050 mg
Vitamin A	36 IU	Vitamin C	62 mg
Vitamin K	0.1 µg		

- Rich in vitamin C.
- Contains phytochemicals—asisothiocyanates, sulforaphane, and indole-3-carbinol. These protect from prostate and colon malignancies.
- Rich in niacin, vitamin B_6, carotenes, vitamin A, vitamin K, thiamin and pantothenic acid.
- Rich in copper, calcium, potassium, manganese, iron, and phosphorus.

LOOFAH SQUASH (Gourd, Luffa, Sponge, Loofa)

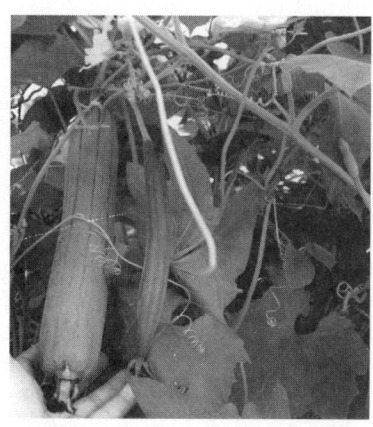

- Very fibrous and low in saturated fat and calories.
- Rich in dietary fiber, vitamin C, riboflavin, zinc, thiamin, iron, and magnesium.
- Contains insulin like peptides, alkaloids that help to reduce blood sugar levels.
- Very low in cholesterol.

TURNIPS

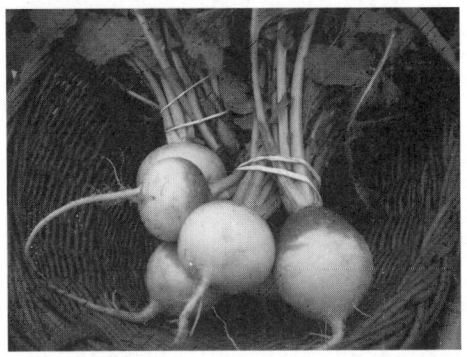

Energy	28 kcal	Carbohydrates	6.43 g
Protein	0.90 g	Fat	0.10 g
Cholesterol	0 mg	Dietary fiber	1.8 g
Sodium	39 mg	Potassium	233 mg
Calcium	30 mg	Copper	0.085 mg
Iron	0.30 mg	Magnesium	11 mg
Manganese	0.134 mg	Zinc	0.27 mg
Folic acid	15 µg	Niacin	0.400 mg
Pantothenic acid	0.200 mg	Pyridoxine	0.090 mg
Riboflavin	0.030 mg	Thiamin	0.040 mg
Vitamin A	0 IU	Vitamin C	21 mg
Vitamin E	0.03 mg	Vitamin K	0.1 µg

- Low calorie root vegetables.
- Rich in vitamin C which prevents from malignancies.
- Rich in folic acid, riboflavin, pyridoxine, pantothenic acid and thiamin.
- Rich in calcium, copper, iron and manganese.

- Boosts up immunity.
- Rich in vitamins A, C, K, carotenoid, xanthin and lutein.

CYPERUS ESCULENTUS (Earth Almond)

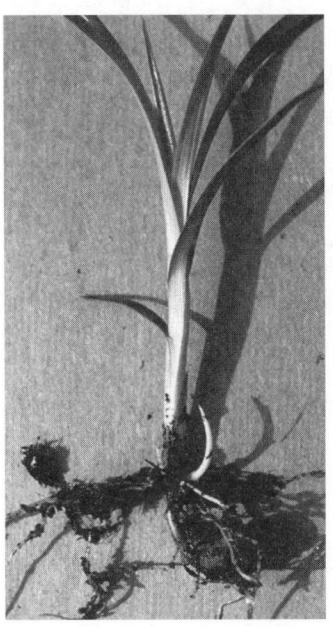

(Per 100 gm)			
Protein	8.6%	Fat	21.8%
Carbohydrate	48%	Magnesium	0.1 mg
Phosphorus	211.5 mg	Potassium	0.5 mg
Starch	33.4 g	Total sugars	14.6 g

"Health" Food

- Prevents heart disease and thrombosis.
- Reduces the risk of colon malignancy.
- Rich in starch, fat, sugar and protein.
- Rich in phosphorus and potassium, vitamins E and C.
- Suitable for diabetics.

SAFFRON

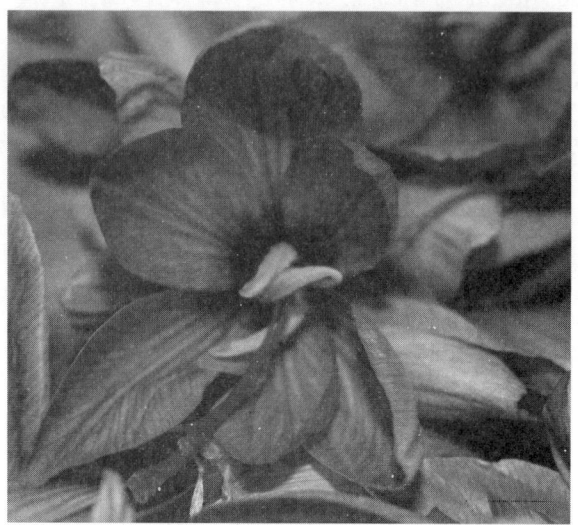

(Per 100 gm)			
Energy	310 kcal	Carbohydrates	65.37 g
Dietary fibre	3.9 g	Fat	5.85 g
Protein	11.43 g	Vitamin A	530 IU
Thiamine	0.115 mg	Riboflavin	0.267 mg
Niacin	1.460 mg	Vitamin C	80.8 mg
Calcium	111 mg	Iron	11.10 mg
Magnesium	264 mg	Phosphorus	252 mg
Potassium	1724 mg	Sodium	148 mg
Zinc	1.09 mg	Selenium	5.6 µg
Folic acid	93 µg	Vitamin B_6	1.010 mg

- World's most costly spices by weight.
- Have anti-carcinogenic, anti-mutagenic, immunomodulating, antioxidant.
- Helps in depression.
- Prevents macular degeneration and retinitis pigmentosa.

CLOVE

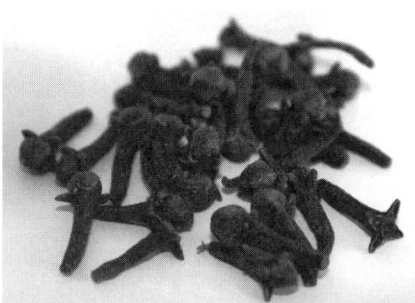

(Per 100 gm)			
Energy	47 kcal	Carbohydrates	10.51 g
Protein	3.27 g	Fat	0.15 g
Cholesterol	0 mg	Dietary fiber	5.4 g
Sodium	94 mg	Potassium	370 mg
Calcium	44 mg	Copper	0.231 mg
Iron	1.28 mg	Magnesium	60 mg
Manganese	0.256 mg	Phosphorus	90 mg
Selenium	7.2 µg	Zinc	2.32 mg
Folic acid	68 µg	Niacin	1.046 mg
Pantothenic acid	0.338 mg	Pyridoxine	0.116 mg
Riboflavin	0.066 mg	Thiamin	0.072 mg
Vitamin A	13 IU	Vitamin C	11.7 mg
Vitamin E	0.19 mg	Vitamin K	14.8 µg

- Good source of proteins, iron, carbohydrates, calcium, phosphorus, potassium, sodium and hydrochloric acid.
- Rich in vitamins A, C, manganese, and dietary fiber.
- Prevents lung malignancy, skin malignancy.
- Useful in treatment of malaria, cholera, scabies and stye.
- Controls blood glucose.
- Prevents bad breath.
- Useful in toothache, sore gums, cold, cough, asthma, bronchitis, sinusitis.
- Acts as antiseptic, antispasmodic agent.

WATERCRESS

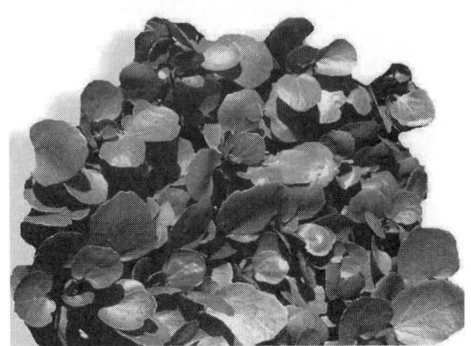

Energy	11 kcal	Carbohydrates	1.29 g
Protein	2.30 g	Fat	0.10 g
Cholesterol	0 mg	Dietary fiber	0.5 g
Sodium	41 mg	Potassium	330 mg
Calcium	120 mg	Copper	0.077 mg
Iron	0.20 mg	Magnesium	21 mg
Manganese	0.244 mg	Phosphorus	60 mg
Selenium	0.9 µg	Zinc	0.11 mg
Folic acid	9 µg	Niacin	0.200 mg
Pantothenic acid	0.310 mg	Pyridoxine	0.129 mg
Riboflavin	0.120 mg	Thiamin	0.090 mg
Vitamin A	3191 IU	Vitamin C	43 mg
Vitamin E	1.0 mg	Vitamin K	250 µg

- Low calorie green leafy vegetables.
- Rich in antioxidants.
- Useful for cholesterol and weight control patients.
- Contains gluconasturtiin-malignancy preventing factor.
- Rich in riboflavin, niacin, vitamin B_6, thiamin and pantothenic.
- Also rich in copper, calcium, potassium, magnesium, manganese and phosphorus.
- Rich in ascorbic acid which boost up immunity.
- Rich in vitamin K which prevents Alzheimer's disease.
- Rich in vitamin A and flavonoids β-carotene, lutein and zeaxanthin.

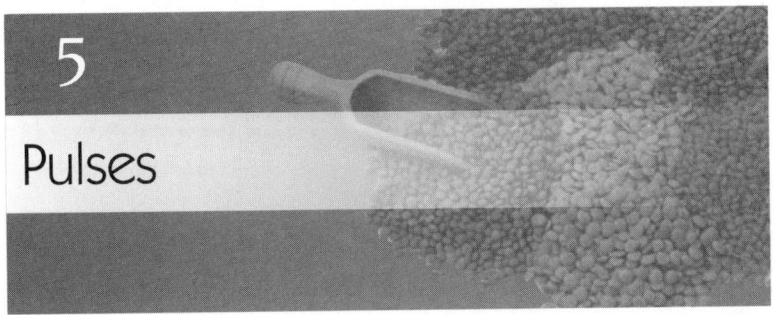

5

Pulses

RED KIDNEY BEANS

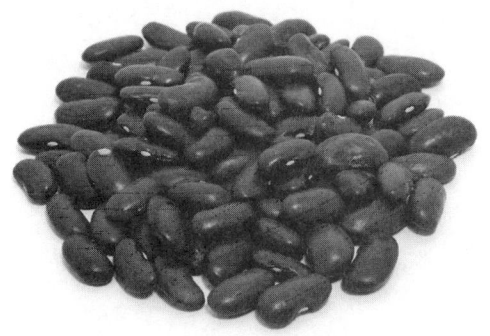

(Per 100 gm)			
Energy	333 kcal	Carbohydrates	60 g
Sugars	2 g	Dietary fiber	15 g
Fat	1 g	Protein	24 g
Calcium	143 mg	Iron	8 mg
Magnesium	140 mg	Potassium	1406 mg
Zinc	3 mg	Pantothenic acid	0.8 mg
Folic acid	394 µg		

- Rich in fiber which prevents constipation.
- Prevents heart disease and rise in cholesterol level.
- Cholesterol free.
- Low sodium which avoid high blood pressure and fluid retention.

- High in iron, magnesium, vitamin C, phosphorus, vitamin A and potassium.
- Rich in folic acid which helps in intrauterine baby to grow and thrive well.
- Very good source of protein.
- Gives more energy to exercise and lose weight.
- Low in fat.

LIMA BEANS

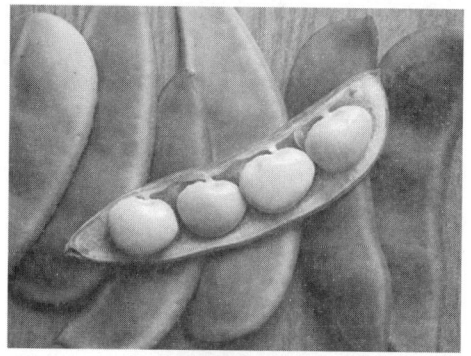

(Per 100 gm)			
Energy	115 kcal	Carbohydrates	20.88 g
Sugars	2.9 g	Dietary fiber	7 g
Fat	0.38 g	Protein	7.8 g
Calcium	17 mg	Iron	2.39 mg
Magnesium	43 mg	Manganese	0.516 mg
Phosphorus	111 mg	Potassium	508 mg
Sodium	2 mg	Zinc	0.95 mg
Thiamine	0.161 mg	Riboflavin	0.055 mg
Niacin	0.421 mg	Pantothenic acid	0.422 mg
Vitamin B_6	0.161 mg	Folic acid	83 µg
Vitamin E	0.18 mg	Vitamin K	2 µg

- Good source of dietary fibre.
- Fat-free.
- Contains high quality protein.

- Contains soluble fibre, which helps regulate blood sugar levels and lowers cholesterol.
- Source of iron.
- Good source of manganese, also molybdenum.
- Contains insoluble fibre which prevents constipation, digestive disorders, irritable bowel syndrome and diverticulitis.
- Good choice for diabetes with insulin resistance.
- Provide folic acid and magnesium.
- Decreases risk factor of heart attack, stroke, and peripheral vascular disease.

AZUKI BEANS, LAL CHAVALI

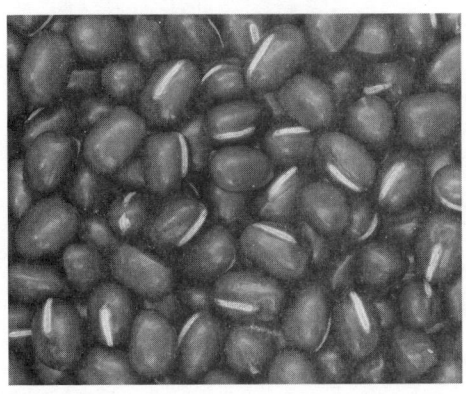

(1 Cup 230 gm)			
Energy	295 kcal	Carbohydrates	56.97 g
Dietary fiber	16.8 g	Fat	0.23 g
Protein	17.3 g	Iron	4.6 mg
Magnesium	120 mg	Phosphorus	386 mg
Potassium	1224 mg	Sodium	18 mg
Zinc	4.07 mg	Thiamine	0.264 mg
Riboflavin	0.147 mg	Niacin	1.649 mg
Pantothenic acid	0.989 mg	Vitamin B_6	0.221 mg
Folic acid	278 µg	Calcium	64 mg

MUNG OR MOONG BEAN

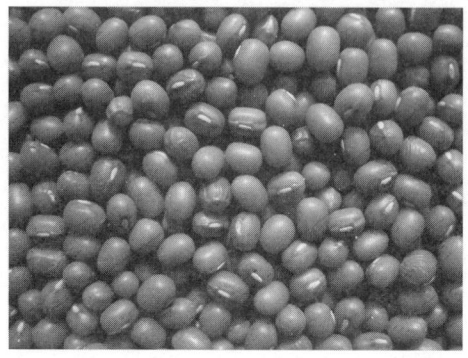

(Per 100 gm Sprouted)		(Per 100 gm Seeds)		(Per 100 gm Boiled)	
Energy	30 kcal	Energy	347 kcal	Energy	105 kcal
Carbohydrates	5.94 g	Carbohydrates	62.62 g	Carbohydrates	19.15 g
Sugars	4.13 g	Sugars	6.6 g	Sugars	2 g
Dietary fiber	1.8 g	Dietary fiber	16.3 g	Dietary fiber	7.6 g
Fat	0.18 g	Fat	1.15 g	Fat	0.38 g
Protein	3.04 g	Protein	23.86 g	Protein	7.02 g
Calcium	13 mg	Calcium	132 mg	Calcium	27 mg
Iron	0.91 mg	Iron	6.74 mg	Iron	1.4 mg
Magnesium	21 mg	Magnesium	189 mg	Magnesium	48 mg
Manganese	0.188 mg	Manganese	1.035 mg	Manganese	0.298 mg
Phosphorus	54 mg	Phosphorus	367 mg	Phosphorus	99 mg
Potassium	149 mg	Potassium	1246 mg	Potassium	266 mg
Zinc	0.41 mg	Zinc	2.68 mg	Zinc	0.84 mg
Thiamine	0.084 mg	Thiamine	0.621 mg	Thiamine	0.164 mg
Riboflavin	0.124 mg	Riboflavin	0.233 mg	Riboflavin	0.061 mg
Niacin	0.749 mg	Niacin	2.251 mg	Niacin	0.577 mg
Pantothenic acid	0.38 mg	Pantothenic acid	1.91 mg	Pantothenic acid	0.41 mg
Vitamin B_6	0.088 mg	Vitamin B_6	0.382 mg	Vitamin B_6	0.067 mg
Folic acid	61 µg	Folic acid	625 µg	Folic acid	159 µg
Vitamin C	13.2 mg	Vitamin C	4.8 mg	Vitamin C	1 mg
Vitamin E	0.1 mg	Vitamin E	0.51 mg	Vitamin E	0.15 mg
Vitamin K	33 µg	Vitamin K	9 µg	Vitamin K	2.7 µg

- Rich in soluble dietary fibers which lowers LDL cholesterol (bad cholesterol).
- Has low glycemic index food which promotes healthy blood sugar levels.
- Best sources of protein.
- Contains protease inhibitors which slows the replication of malignancy cells in breast.
- Contains phytoestrogen which relieves hot flashes in post-menopausal women.

VIGNA MUNGO, BLACK GRAM-URAD DAL

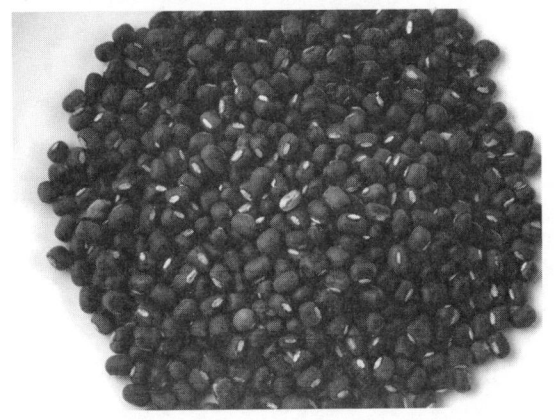

Energy	341 cal	Protein	24%
Fat	1.4%	Carbohydrates	59.6%
Calcium	154 mg	Phosphorous	385 mg
Iron	9.1 mg		

- Have immunostimulatory activity.
- Rich in potassium, phosphorus, calcium and sodium.
- Rich in vitamins A, B_1 and B_3.
- Also have thiamine, riboflavin, niacin, vitamin C and iron.
- Useful in diabetes, sexual dysfunction, nervous disorders, hair disorders, digestive system disorders and rheumatic afflictions.

PHASEOLUS COCCINEUS (Runner Bean)

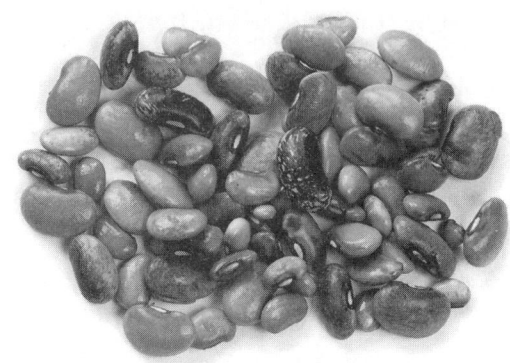

(Per 100 gm)			
Energy	338 kcal	Protein	20.3 gm
Fat	1.8 gm	Carbohydrate	62.0 gm
Fibre	4.8 gm	Calcium	114 mg
Phosphorus	354 mg	Iron	9.0 mg
Thiamin	0.50 mg	Riboflavin	0.19 mg
Niacin	2.3 mg	Ascorbic acid	2 mg

VIGNA UMBELLATA (Rice Bean)

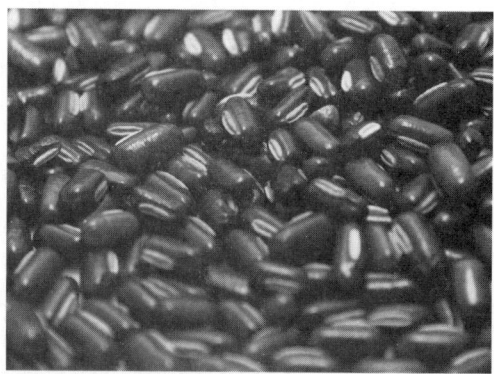

- Protein 25.57%.
- Rich in unsaturated fatty-linoleic and linolenic acids.

VIGNA ACONITIFOLIUS (Moth Bean or मटकी)

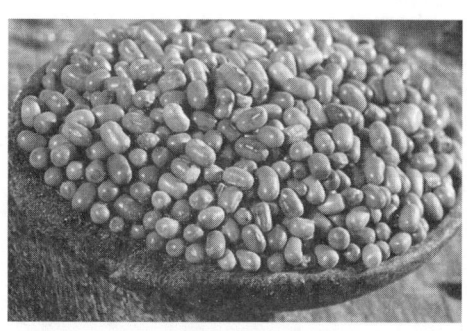

(Per 100 gm)			
Sprouted:		**Seeds:**	
Energy	250 kcal	Energy	330 cal
Sodium	227 mg	Moisture	11 gm
Fat	6 g	Protein	24 gm
Saturated	1 g	Fat	1 gm
Carbohydrates	37 g	Mineral	3 gm
Polyunsaturated	1 g	Fibre	4 gm
Dietary fiber	0 g	Carbohydrates	56 gm
Monounsaturated	4 g	Calcium	202 mg
Protein	14 g	Phosphorous	230 mg
Cholesterol	0 mg	Iron	9 mg

PHASEOLUS ACUTIFOLIUS (Brown Beans)

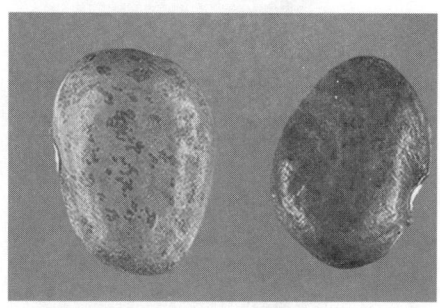

(Per ½ cup)					
Calories	360	Potassium	1690 mg	Dietary fiber	43 grams

- High in fiber.
- Low glycemic index.
- Rich in calcium, iron, magnesium, zinc, phosphorus, and potassium.
- Low in polyunsaturated fat.
- Gluten free.
- Ideal for diabetes.
- Controls blood sugar levels.
- Rich in protein.

FAVA BEANS

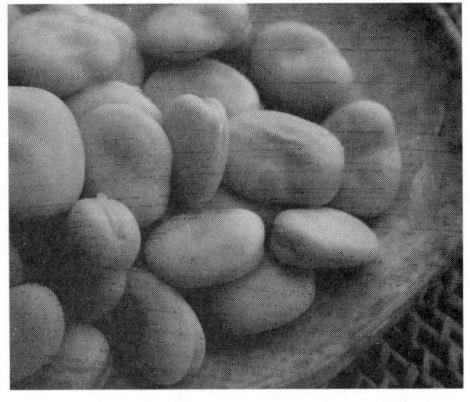

(Per 100 gm)			
Energy	341 kcal	Carbohydrates	58.29 g
Dietary fiber	25 g	Fat	1.53 g
Protein	26.12 g	Calcium	103 mg
Iron	6.7 mg	Magnesium	192 mg
Manganese	1.626 mg	Phosphorus	421 mg
Potassium	1062 mg	Sodium	13 mg
Zinc	3.14 mg	Thiamine	0.555 mg
Riboflavin	0.333 mg	Niacin	2.832 mg
Vitamin B_6	0.366 mg	Folic acid	423 µg
Vitamin C	1.4 mg	Vitamin K	9 µg

- Contains vicine and convicine which induce hemolytic anemia in patients with the hereditary condition glucose-6-phosphate dehydrogenase deficiency (Favism).
- Rich in L-DOPA which is helpful in treatment of Parkinson's disease and hypertension.

PEAS GREEN

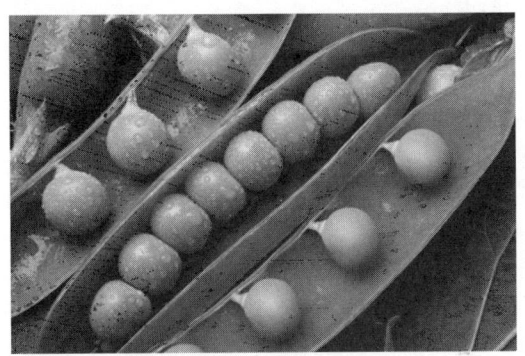

(Per 100 gm)			
Energy	81 kcal	Carbohydrates	14.45 g
Sugars	5.67 g	Dietary fiber	5.1 g
Fat	0.4 g	Protein	5.42 g
Vitamin A	38 µg	Beta-carotene	449 µg
Thiamine	0.266 mg	Riboflavin	0.132 mg
Niacin	2.09 mg	Vitamin B_6	0.169 mg
Folic acid	65 µg	Vitamin C	40 mg
Vitamin E	0.13 mg	Vitamin K	24.8 µg
Calcium	25 mg	Iron	1.47 mg
Magnesium	33 mg	Manganese	0.41 mg
Phosphorus	108 mg	Potassium	244 mg
Sodium	5 mg	Zinc	1.24 mg

- Low in calories.
- Good source of proteins.
- Rich in soluble as well as insoluble fiber.
- Excellent source of folic acid which prevents neural tube defects in the newborn babies.

- Rich in antioxidants flavonoids such as carotenes, lutein and zeaxanthin as well as vitamin A.
- Protects from lung and oral cavity malignancies.
- Rich in pantothenic acid, niacin, thiamin, folic acid and pyridoxine.
- Rich in calcium, iron, copper, zinc, and manganese.
- Very good in ascorbic acid—powerful natural water-soluble antioxidant.
- Contains phytosterols-β-sitosterol which helps to lower cholesterol levels in the body.
- Rich in vitamin K which has role in Alzheimer's disease.

CHICKPEAS (Ghana/Bengal Gram)

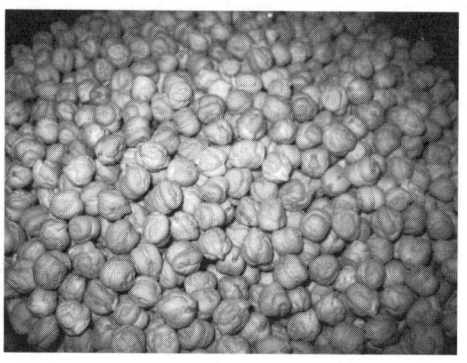

(Per 100 gm)			
Energy	164 kcal	Carbohydrates	27.42 g
Sugars	4.8 g	Dietary fiber	7.6 g
Fat	2.59 g	Protein	8.86 g
Calcium	49 mg	Iron	2.89 mg
Magnesium	48 mg	Phosphorus	168 mg
Potassium	291 mg	Sodium	7 mg
Zinc	1.53 mg	Vitamin A	1 µg
Thiamine	0.116 mg	Riboflavin	0.063 mg
Niacin	0.526 mg	Pantothenic acid	0.286 mg
Vitamin B_6	0.139 mg	Folic acid	172 µg
Vitamin B_{12}	0 µg	Vitamin C	1.3 mg
Vitamin E	0.35 mg	Vitamin K	4 µg

- Rich in zinc, folic acid and protein.
- Low in fat-polyunsaturated.
- Fibre content higher.
- Rich in Phosphorus.
- Low in cholesterol.

LENTIL/MASOOR DAL

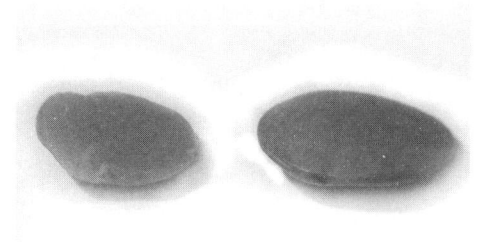

(Per 100 gm)			
Energy	353 kcal	Carbohydrates	60 g
Sugars	2 g	Dietary fiber	31 g
Fat	1 g	Protein	26 g
Calcium	56 mg	Iron	7.54 mg
Magnesium	122 mg	Phosphorus	451 mg
Potassium	955 mg	Sodium	6 mg
Zinc	4.78 mg	Thiamine	0.87 mg
Riboflavin	0.211 mg	Niacin	2.605 mg
Pantothenic acid	2.120 mg	Vitamin B_6	0.54 mg
Folic acid	479 µg	Vitamin C	4.4 mg

- Third-highest level of protein, after soybeans and hemp.
- High levels of slowly digested starch.
- Rich in iron.
- Proteins include the essential amino acids isoleucine and lysine.
- Contains dietary fiber, folic acid, vitamin B_1, and minerals.

PEANUTS (Arachis Hypogaea)

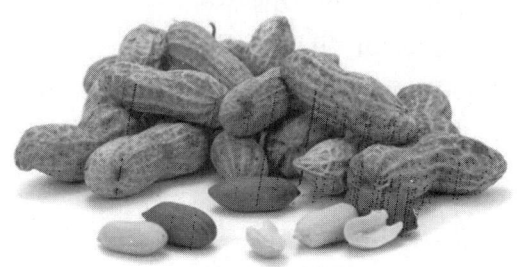

(Per 100 gm)			
Energy	567 kcal	Carbohydrates	16.13 g
Protein	25.80 g	Fat	49.24 g
Cholesterol	0 mg	Dietary fiber	8.5 g
Sodium	18 mg	Potassium	705 mg
Calcium	92 mg	Copper	1.144 mg
Iron	4.58 mg	Magnesium	168 mg
Manganese	1.934 mg	Phosphorus	76 mg
Selenium	7.2 µg	Zinc	3.27 mg
Folic acid	240 µg	Niacin	12.066 mg
Pantothenic acid	1.767 mg	Pyridoxine	0.348 mg
Riboflavin	0.135 mg	Thiamin	0.640 mg
Vitamin A	0 IU	Vitamin C	0
Vitamin E	8.33 mg		

- Rich in energy.
- Adequate in mono-unsaturated fatty acids—oleic acid.
- Helps to lower bad cholesterol and increases good cholesterol.
- Prevent coronary artery disease and strokes.
- Rich source of copper, manganese, potassium, calcium, iron, magnesium, zinc and selenium.
- Useful in hemophilia, nose bleeding, reducing excessive menstruation bleeding in women.
- Rich in protein which are essential for growth and development.

- Contains resveratrol-polyphenolics antioxidant which have against malignancies, heart disease, degenerative nerve disease, and Alzheimer's disease.
- Excellent source of vitamin E—a powerful lipid soluble antioxidant.
- Rich in riboflavin, niacin, thiamin, pantothenic acid, vitamin B_6, and folic acid.

WINGED BEAN PEA

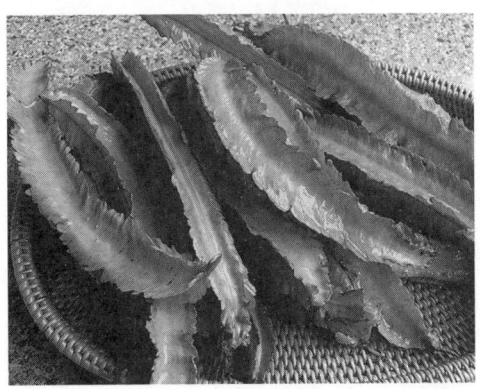

(Per 100 gm)			
Energy	409 kcal	Carbohydrates	41.7 g
Dietary fiber	25.9 g	Fat	16.3 g
Protein	29.65 g	Calcium	440 mg
Iron	13.44 mg	Magnesium	179 mg
Manganese	3.721 mg	Phosphorus	451 mg
Potassium	977 mg	Sodium	38 mg
Zinc	4.48 mg	Thiamine	1.03 mg
Riboflavin	0.45 mg	Niacin	3.09 mg
Pantothenic acid	0.795 mg	Vitamin B_6	0.175 mg
Folic acid	45 µg		

- Richer in protein.
- Good source of vitamins A, C, calcium and iron.

SWORD BEANS

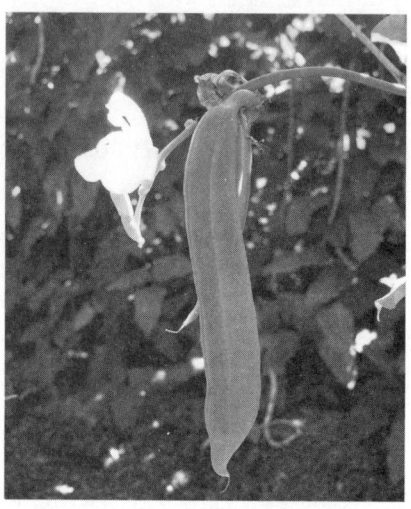

Energy	44 kcal	Protein	3 gm
Fat	0 gm	Mineral	1 gm
Fibre	1 gm	Carbohydrates	8 gm
Calcium	60 mg	Phosphorous	40 mg
Iron	2 mg		

PIGEON PEAS (Toor Dal)

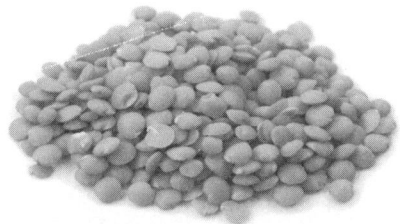 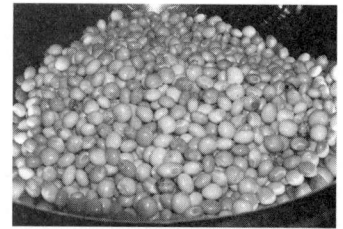

Split (per 100 gm)		*Raw (per 100 gm)*	
Energy	343 kcal	Energy	136 kcal
Carbohydrates	62.78 g	Carbohydrates	23.88 g
Dietary fiber	15 g	Sugars	3 g

(*contd.*)

(contd.)

Split (per 100 gm)		Raw (per 100 gm)	
Energy	343 kcal	Energy	136 kcal
Carbohydrates	62.78 g	Carbohydrates	23.88 g
Dietary fiber	15 g	Sugars	3 g
Fat	1.49 g	Dietary fiber	5.1 g
Protein	21.7 g	Fat	1.64 g
Calcium	130 mg	Protein	7.2 g
Iron	5.23 mg	Calcium	42 mg
Magnesium	183 mg	Iron	1.6 mg
Manganese	1.791 mg	Magnesium	68 mg
Phosphorus	367 mg	Manganese	0.574 mg
Potassium	1392 mg	Phosphorus	127 mg
Sodium	17 mg	Potassium	552 mg
Zinc	2.76 mg	Sodium	5 mg
Thiamine	0.643 mg	Zinc	1.04 mg
Riboflavin	0.187 mg	Thiamine	0.4 mg
Niacin	2.965 mg	Riboflavin	0.17 mg
Pantothenic acid	1.266 mg	Niacin	2.2 mg
Vitamin B_6	0.283 mg	Pantothenic acid	0.68 mg
Folic acid	456 µg	Vitamin B_6	0.068 mg
		Folic acid	173 µg
		Vitamin C	39 mg
		Vitamin E	0.39 mg
		Vitamin K	24 µg

BLACK-EYED PEA

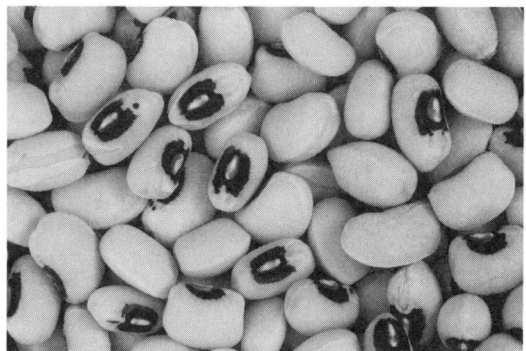

(Per 100 gm)			
Energy	116 kcal	Carbohydrates	20.76 g
Sugars	3.3 g	Dietary fiber	6.5 g
Fat	0.53 g	Protein	7.73 g
Calcium	24 mg	Iron	2.51 mg
Magnesium	53 mg	Manganese	0.475 mg
Phosphorus	156 mg	Potassium	278 mg
Sodium	4 mg	Zinc	1.29 mg
Thiamine	0.202 mg	Riboflavin	0.055 mg
Niacin	0.495 mg	Pantothenic acid	0.411 mg
Vitamin B_6	0.1 mg	Folic acid	208 µg
Vitamin E	0.28 mg	Vitamin K	1.7 µg

KIDNEY BEANS RAJMAH

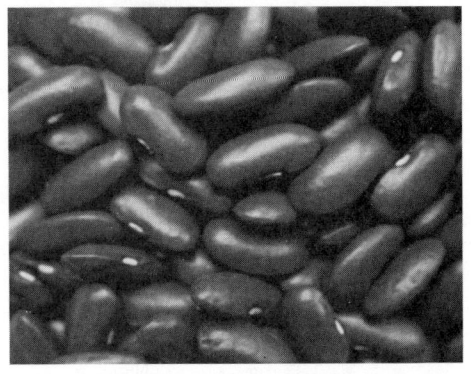

Energy	346 kcal	Moisture	12 gm
Protein	23 gm	Fat	1 gm
Mineral	3 gm	Fibre	5 gm
Carbohydrates	61 gm	Calcium	260 mg
Phosphorous	410 mg	Iron	5 mg

- High in folic acid, protein and mineral content.
- Helps to lower the homocysteine levels in the body.
- Rich in soluble and insoluble fiber.
- Rich in iron and magnesium.
- Low in calories.

- Fat-free.
- Prevents digestive disorders like irritable bowel syndrome.

SOYA BEAN

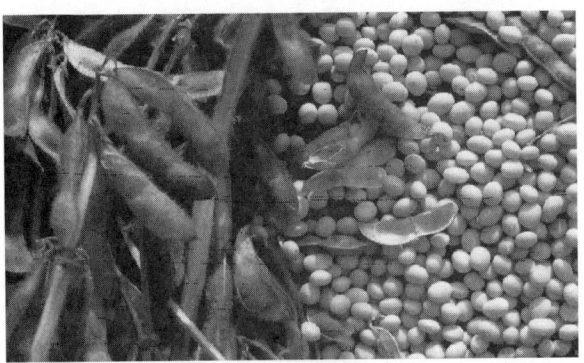

(Per 100 gm)			
Energy	446 kcal	Carbohydrates	30.16 g
Sugars	7.33 g	Dietary fiber	9.3 g
Fat	19.94 g	Protein	36.49 g
Calcium	277 mg	Iron	15.7 mg
Magnesium	280 mg	Manganese	2.517 mg
Phosphorus	704 mg	Potassium	1797 mg
Sodium	2 mg	Zinc	4.89 mg
Vitamin A	1 μg	Thiamine	0.874 mg
Riboflavin	0.87 mg	Niacin	1.623 mg
Pantothenic acid	0.793 mg	Vitamin B_6	0.377 mg
Folic acid	375 μg	Choline	115.9 mg
Vitamin C	6.0 mg	Vitamin E	0.85 mg
Vitamin K	47 μg		

- Complete source of protein and essential amino acids.
- Safe for breast malignancy.
- Improvement in cognitive function, particularly verbal memory and in frontal lobe function.
- Rich in omega-3 fatty acid alpha-linolenic acid which prevents malignancies.
- Lowers bad cholesterol.

ALFALFA SEED—SPROUTED

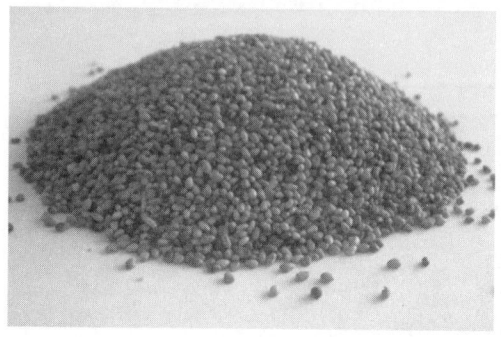

(Per 100 gm)			
Energy	23 kcal	Carbohydrates	2.1 g
Dietary fiber	1.9 g	Fat	0.7 g
Protein	4 g	Calcium	32 mg
Iron	0.96 mg	Magnesium	27 mg
Manganese	0.188 mg	Phosphorus	70 mg
Potassium	79 mg	Sodium	6 mg
Zinc	0.92 mg	Thiamine	0.076 mg
Riboflavin	0.126 mg	Niacin	0.481 mg
Pantothenic acid	0.563 mg	Vitamin B$_6$	0.034 mg
Folic acid	36 µg	Vitamin C	8.2 mg
Vitamin K	30.5 µg		

OATS

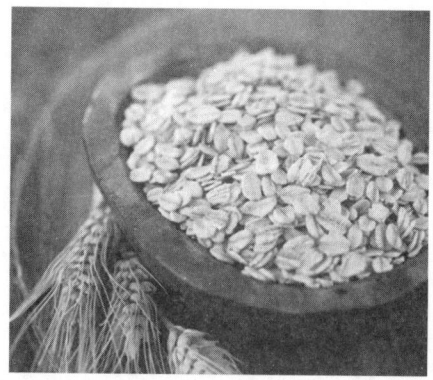

(Per 100 g)			
Energy	389 kcal	Carbohydrates	66.3 g
Dietary fibre	10.6 g	Fat	6.9 g
Protein	16.9 g	Calcium	54 mg
Iron	5 mg	Magnesium	177 mg
Manganese	4.9 mg	Phosphorus	523 mg
Potassium	429 mg	Zinc	4 mg
Thiamine	0.763 mg	Riboflavin	0.139 mg
Niacin	0.961 mg	Pantothenic acid	1.349 mg
Folic acid	56 µg		

- Healthy food.
- Gluten-free.
- Has cholesterol-lowering properties.
- Reduces the risk of heart disease.
- Rich in soluble fiber which helps in digestion and an extended sensation of fullness.
- Rich in lipid and protein.

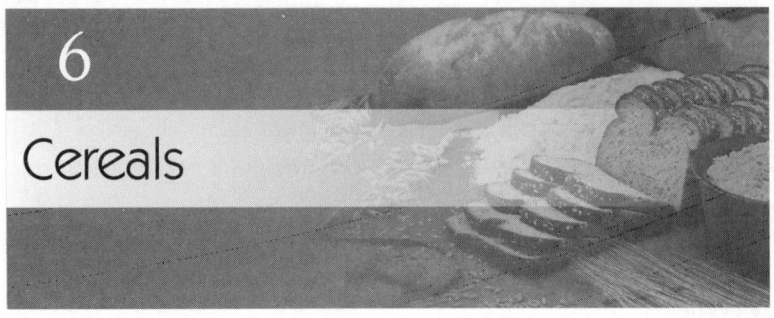

6

Cereals

WHEAT

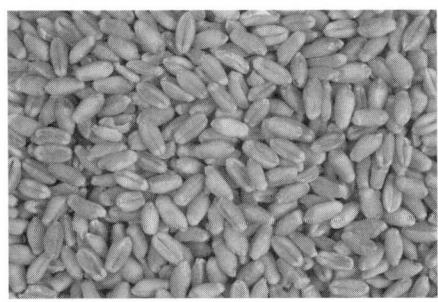

(Per 100 gm)			
Energy	327 kcal	Carbohydrates	71.18 g
Sugars	0.41 g	Dietary fiber	12.2 g
Fat	1.54 g	Protein	12.61 g
Calcium	29 mg	Iron	3.19 mg
Magnesium	126 mg	Manganese	3.985 mg
Phosphorus	288 mg	Potassium	363 mg
Sodium	2 mg	Zinc	2.65 mg
Thiamine	0.383 mg	Riboflavin	0.115 mg
Niacin	5.464 mg	Pantothenic acid	0.954 mg
Vitamin B_6	0.3 mg	Folic acid	38 µg
Vitamin E	1.01 mg	Vitamin K	1.9 µg

- Rich in carbohydrates.
- Rich in manganese, phosphorus, magnesium and selenium.
- Rich in zinc, copper, iron and potassium.

- Rich in vitamin B_6, niacin, thiamin, folic acid, riboflavin and pantothenic acid.
- Prevents from heart diseases, osteoporosis, Alzheimer's diseases, and type-2 diabetes.
- Rich in gluten, so should be avoided by people suffering from gluten intolerance.
- Wheat allergy.
- Contains vitamins E and K.
- Rich in protein.
- Controls obesity.
- Preventing type-2 diabetes, gallstones.
- Protection against breast malignancy.
- Prevents childhood asthma.
- It is source of betaine which aids in preventing chronic inflammation.

Whole Wheat

- Reduces the risk of metabolic syndrome.
- Preventing visceral obesity.
- Low levels of protective HDL cholesterol.
- High triglycerides.
- High blood pressure.
- Reduces the risk of heart diseases.
- Regulating blood glucose in diabetes.

BRAN (Miller's Bran)

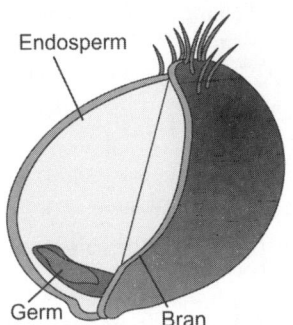

Endosperm

Germ   Bran

Nutrients (%)	Wheat	Rye	Oat	Rice	Barley
Carbohydrates	45–50	50–70	16–34	18–23	70–80
Starch	13–18	12–15	18–45	18–30	8–11
Proteins	15–18	8–9	13–20	15–18	11–15
Fats	4–5	4–5	6–11	18–23	1–2

- Hard outer layers of cereal grain.
- It consists of the combined aleurone and pericarp.

WHEAT GERM

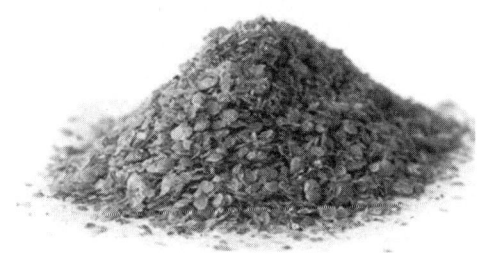

(Per 100 gm)			
Energy	382 kcal	Carbohydrates	51.8 g
Sugars	7.8 g	Dietary fiber	15.1 g
Fat	10.7 g	Saturated	1.83 g
Monounsaturated	1.5 g	Polyunsaturated	6.62 g
Protein	29.1 g	Calcium	45 mg
Iron	9.09 mg	Magnesium	320 mg
Manganese	19.956 mg	Phosphorus	1146 mg
Potassium	947 mg	Zinc	16.67 mg
Thiamine	1.67 mg	Riboflavin	0.82 mg
Niacin	5.59 mg	Pantothenic acid	1.387 mg
Vitamin B_6	0.978 mg	Folic acid	352 µg
Vitamin C	6 mg	Vitamin E	15.99 mg

- Healthy food.
- Rich in fiber—important for prevention of colon malignancy.
- Rich in zinc, vitamin E, B complex vitamins, proteins and unsaturated fat.
- Contains an antioxidant which boost up body's immune system.

- Rich in folic acid which prevents neural-tube birth defects.
- Contains a phytonutrient L-ergothioneine, a powerful anti-oxidant.
- Useful for athletes and body builders which improves cardio-vascular function and endurance levels.

JOWAR

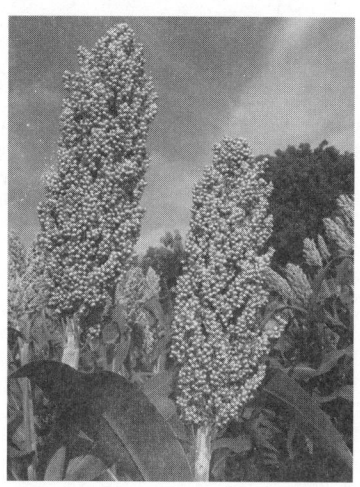

Energy	349 cal	Moisture	12 gm
Protein	10 gm	Fat	2 gm
Mineral	2 gm	Fibre	2 gm
Carbohydrates	73 gm	Calcium	25 gm
Phosphorous	222 gm	Iron	4 mg

- Rich in fiber which lowers risk of obesity, stroke, high blood pressure, heart disease, diabetes, blood cholesterol, diverticular disease and colon malignancy, constipation and hemorrhoids.
- Iron present is non-heme iron, a form of the mineral that is not absorbed.
- Rich in phosphorus and thiamine.
- Prevents heart failure, Alzheimer's disease and cataracts.

BAJRA

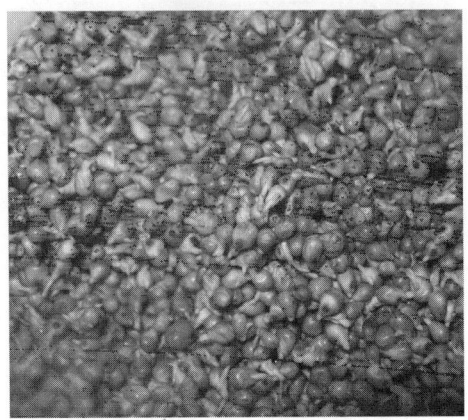

(Per 100 gm)			
Energy	361 cal	Moisture	12 gm
Protein	12 gm	Fat	5 gm
Mineral	2 gm	Fibre	1 gm
Carbohydrates	67 gm	Calcium	42 mg
Phosphorous	296 mg	Iron	8 mg

- Eating bajra with honey in the morning are very effective for bleeding piles, epilepsy, insomnia, impotency, high blood pressure, diabetes and tuberculosis.
- Rich in fiber so good for diabetics.
- Rich in fiber so useful for weight loss.
- Maintains cardiovascular.
- Controls blood sugar levels.
- Easily digestible.
- Lower allergic reactions.
- Gluten free—useful for celiac disease.
- Helpful for severe constipation and stomach ulcers.
- Contains phytic acid and niacin which helps in lowering the cholesterol.

SWEET CORN

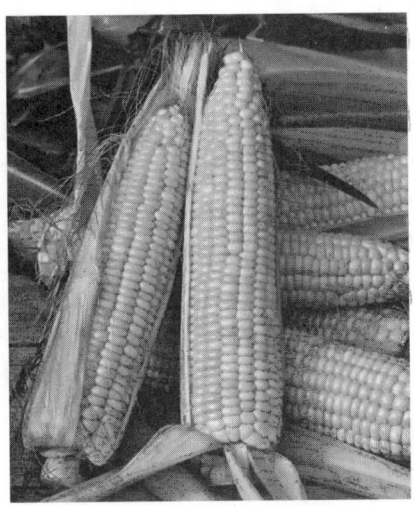

(Per 100 gm)			
Energy	86 kcal	Carbohydrates	18.7 g
Starch	5.7 g	Sugars	6.26 g
Dietary fiber	2 g	Fat	1.35 g
Protein	3.27 g	Iron	0.52 mg
Magnesium	37 mg	Manganese	0.163 mg
Phosphorus	89 mg	Potassium	270 mg
Zinc	0.46 mg	Vitamin A	9 µg
Thiamine	0.155 mg	Riboflavin	0.055 mg
Niacin	1.77 mg	Pantothenic acid	0.717 mg
Vitamin B_6	0.093 mg	Folic acid	42 µg
Vitamin C	6.8 mg		

- Rich in B vitamins, folic acid, vitamin C, beta-carotene, protein and fiber.
- It also contains an abundance of carbohydrates,
- High sugar content.
- Have anti-malignancy properties.

OAT

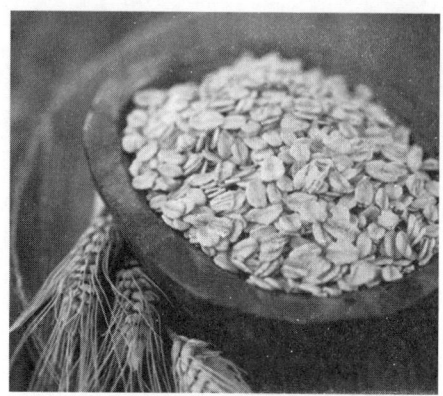

	(Per 100 gm)		
Energy	389 kcal	Carbohydrates	66.3 g
Dietary fibre	10.6 g	Fat	6.9 g
Protein	16.9 g	Calcium	54 mg
Iron	5 mg	Magnesium	177 mg
Manganese	4.9 mg	Phosphorus	523 mg
Potassium	429 mg	Zinc	4 mg
Thiamine	0.763 mg	Riboflavin	0.139 mg
Niacin	0.961 mg	Pantothenic acid	1.349 mg
Folic acid	56 µg		

- Healthy food.
- Good source of thiamin, folic acid, biotin, pantothenic acid and vitamin E.
- Rich in zinc, selenium, copper, iron, manganese and magnesium. Lowers bad cholesterol so decrease risk of heart disease.
- Reduce hypertension.
- Rich in soluble and insoluble fiber. So relieving constipation.
- Decreased risk of obesity.
- Useful for weight reduction because of slower digestion and an extended sensation of fullness.
- Sustained rise in blood sugars over a longer time period.
- Rich in phytochemicals which decrease the risk of breast, prostate, endometrial and ovarian malignancy.

ELEUSINE CORACANA—FINGER MILLET/ RAGI

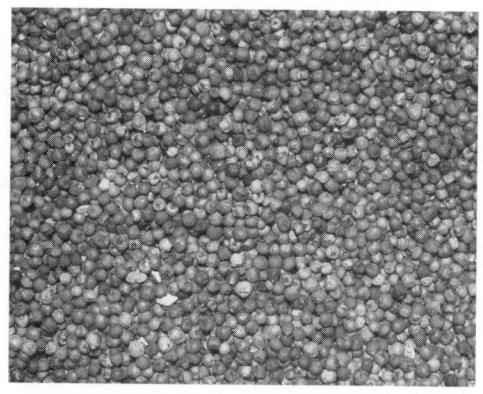

Energy	328 kcal	Moisture	13 gm
Protein	7 gm	Fat	1 gm
Mineral	3 gm	Fibre	4 gm
Carbohydrates	72 gm	Calcium	344 mg
Phosphorous	283 mg	Iron	4 mg

- Rich source of calcium, iron and protein.
- Low in unsaturated fat.
- Gluten free.
- Most nutritious cereals.
- Contains tryptophan which lowers appetite and keeps weight in control.
- Prevents anxiety, migraines, depression and insomnia.
- Prevents malnutrition, degenerative diseases and premature aging.
- Green ragi is useful in lactating mother for milk production.
- Rich in calcium which helps in strengthening bones.
- Contains phytochemicals which helps in slowing digestion process, controlling blood sugar.
- Contains lecithin and methionine which brings down cholesterol level.
- Rich in natural iron.

AMARANTH GRAIN—RAJGIRA

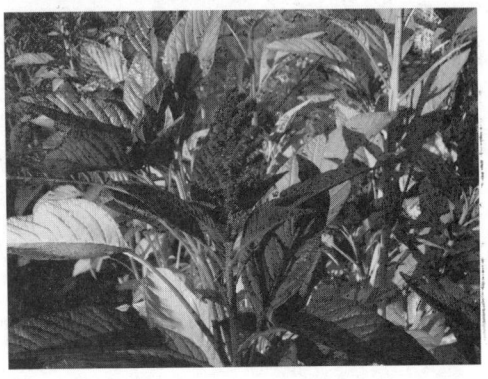

(Per 100 gm)			
Energy	371 kcal	Carbohydrates	65 g
Sugars	1.7 g	Dietary fiber	7 g
Fat	7 g	Protein	14 g
Calcium	159 mg	Iron	7.6 mg
Magnesium	248 mg	Manganese	3.4 mg
Phosphorus	557 mg	Potassium	508 mg
Zinc	2.9 mg	Thiamine	0.1 mg
Riboflavin	0.2 mg	Niacin	0.9 mg
Pantothenic acid	1.5 mg	Vitamin B$_6$	0.6 mg
Folic acid	82 µg		

- Supernatural.
- Good source of vitamin A, vitamin B$_6$, vitamin K, vitamin C, folic acid and riboflavin.
- Rich in calcium, potassium, iron, copper, magnesium, phosphorus and manganese.
- Useful for energy production, glossy nails and glowing skin, prevention of muscle cramps and spasms, elasticity of body tissues, maintenance of blood sugar levels and healthy hair. Decreases depression and anxiety.
- Rich in protein—contains a complete set of amino acids.
- Gluten free.
- Dietary fiber and lysine which is helpful in malignancy treatment.

- Low in cholesterol.
- Prevents hypertension and cardiovascular disease.
- Boost up immune system.
- Prevention of premature greying of the hair.
- Rich in vitamin B_6, folic acid, niacin, riboflavin and pantothenic acid.

RYE-TRITICEAE

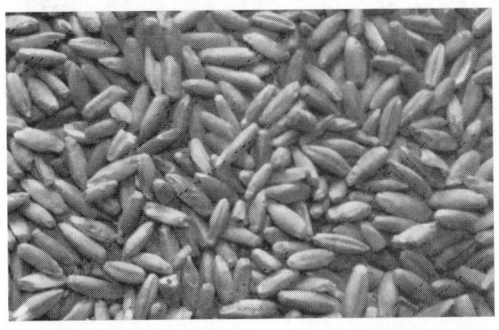

(Per 100 gm)			
Energy	335 calories	Calcium	33 mg
Iron	2.67 mg	Manganese	121 mg
Phosphorus	374 mg	Potassium	264 mg
Sodium	6 mg	Zinc	3.73 mg
Copper	0.450 mg	Magnesium	2.680 mg
Selenium	0.035 mg		

- Rye is rich in potassium, phosphorus and magnesium.
- Good amount of calcium, sodium, iron, zinc, copper, manganese and selenium.
- Rich in choline, vitamins A, B_6, niacin, thiamin, riboflavin and pantothenic acid.
- Lowers the risk of Type II diabetes, reduces high blood pressure.
- Good for postmenopausal women with high cholesterol.
- Helps in reducing weight.
- Prevents gallstones, heart failure, breast malignancy and childhood asthma.

BUCKWHEAT

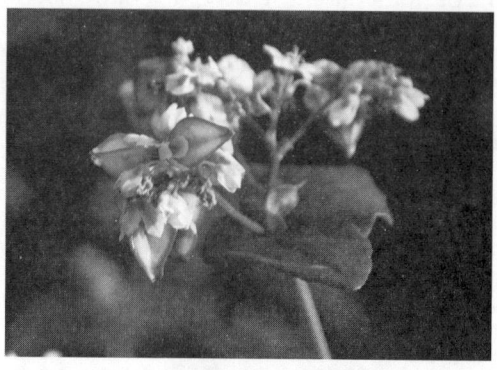

Starch 71–78%

Crude protein is 18%

Rich in all essential amino acids—lysine, threonine, tryptophan

- Grain in the himalayas.
- High in protein.
- Reduces plasma cholesterol, body fat and gallstones.

FONIO

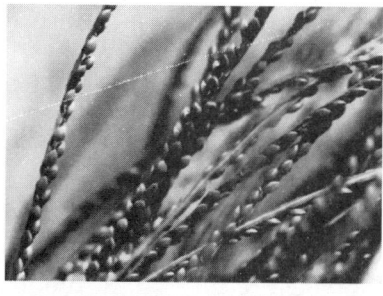

Proteins	8–10%	Carbohydrates	85%
Sugars	85%	Protein	10%
Fat	3, 5%		
Rich in sulphur			

- Grown in West Africa.
- Highly rich in amino acids and iron.
- Vital role in nourishing human health.
- Nutritious for pregnant women and children.
- Free of gluten.
- Rich in calcium, magnesium, zinc and manganese.
- Contains high levels of methionine and cystine, amino acids.

QUINOA

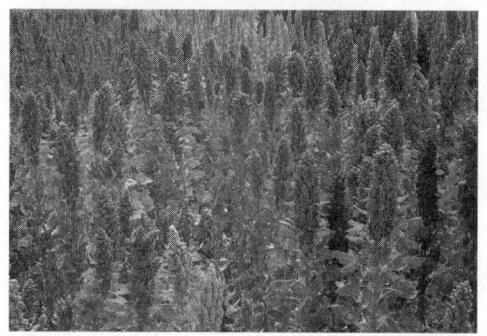

	(Per 100 gm)		
Energy	368 kcal	Carbohydrates	64 g
Starch	52 g	Dietary fibre	7 g
Fat	6 g	Protein	14 g
Calcium	36 mg	Iron	4.6 mg
Magnesium	197 mg	Phosphorus	457 mg
Potassium	563 mg	Zinc	3.1 mg
Thiamine	0.36 mg	Riboflavin	0.32 mg
Vitamin B_6	0.5 mg	Folic acid	184 µg

- Super food.
- Source of complete protein.
- Good source of dietary fiber and phosphorus.
- High in magnesium and iron.
- Source of calcium.
- Gluten-free.

TRITICALE

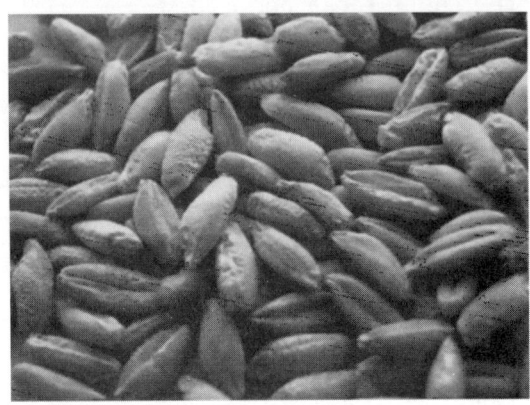

(Per 100 gm)			
Calories	336 cal	Fat	2.1 g
Saturated fat	0.4 g	Polyunsaturated fat	0.9 g
Monounsaturated fat	0.2 g	Cholesterol	0 mg
Sodium	5 mg	Potassium	332 mg
Carbohydrateohydrate	72 g	Protein	13 g

- A hybrid of wheat and rye.
- First bred in laboratories during the late 19th century.
- The grain was originally bred in Scotland and Sweden.

RICE

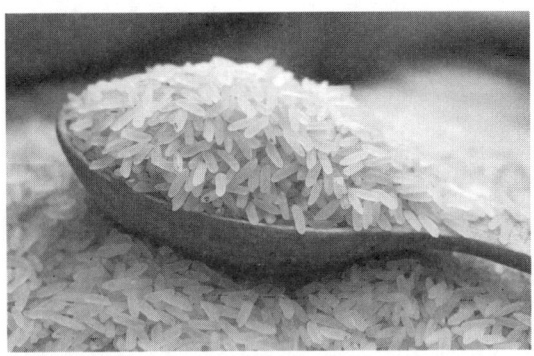

(Per 100 gm)			
Energy	365 kcal	Carbohydrates	80 g
Sugars	0.12 g	Dietary fiber	1.3 g
Fat	0.66 g	Protein	7.13 g
Calcium	28 mg	Iron	0.80 mg
Magnesium	25 mg	Manganese	1.088 mg
Phosphorus	115 mg	Potassium	115 mg
Zinc	1.09 mg	Thiamine	0.0701 mg
Riboflavin	0.0149 mg	Niacin	1.62 mg
Pantothenic acid	1.014 mg	Vitamin B_6	0.164 mg

- Staple food for half the world's population.
- Rich in carbohydrates.
- Great source of energy.
- Cholesterol free.
- Rich in insoluble fiber that protects against malignancies esp. colorectal and intestinal.
- Rich in natural antioxidants like vitamins C, A, phenolic and flavonoid compounds.
- Cool off inflamed skin surfaces.
- Delay the appearance of wrinkles and prevents Alzheimer's diseases.
- Low levels of fat, cholesterol, and sodium help to reduce obesity.
- Low in sodium.
- Best foods for hypertensives.
- Effective medicine for dysentery.
- Have diuretic properties.
- As per Chinese, it increases appetite.
- Bowel movement regularity.
- Excellent source of niacin, vitamin D, calcium, fiber, iron, thiamine and riboflavin.
- Rice bran oil promotes cardiovascular strength by reducing cholesterol.
- Rich in resistant starch which is helpful in irritable bowel syndrome and diarrhea.
- Prevents chronic constipation.
- Brown rice is beneficial for normal functioning of the nervous system and the production of sex hormones.

RICE BRAN

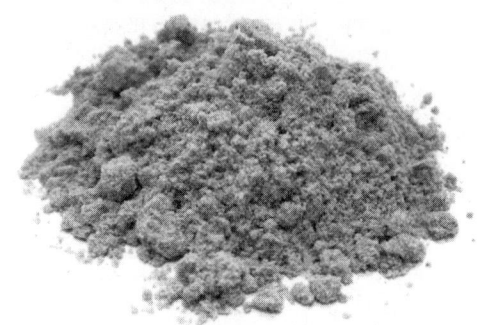

Energy	393 kcal	Moisture	11 gm
Protein	13 gm	Fat	16 gm
Mineral	7 gm	Fibre	4 gm
Carbohydrates	48 gm	Calcium	67 mg
Phosphorous	1410 mg	Iron	35 mg

- "Wonder food."
- Excellent source of amino acids for muscle building, carbohydrates for energy, fiber for maintaining healthy circulation and digestion, and vitamins and minerals for the growth and health of cells.
- Rich in antioxidants useful against malignancy and aging.
- No cholesterol or trans fat.
- Rich in dietary fiber which lowers cholesterol.
- Rich in vitamins B complex and E, good source of phosphorus, zinc, potassium, magnesium and manganese.
- Gluten free.
- Lactose free.
- Hypoallergenic.
- Low glycemic index (<50).
- Great weight loss management.
- Helps burn fat.

RICE-FLAKES

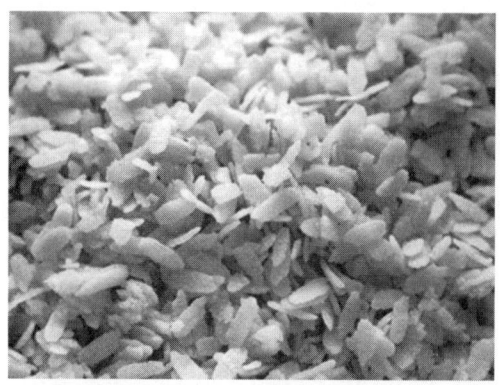

Energy	346 kcal	Moisture	12 gm
Protein	7 gm	Fat	1 gm
Mineral	2 gm	Fibre	1 gm
Carbohydrates	77 gm	Calcium	20 mg
Phosphorous	238 mg	Iron	20 mg

RICE-PARBOILED-MILLED

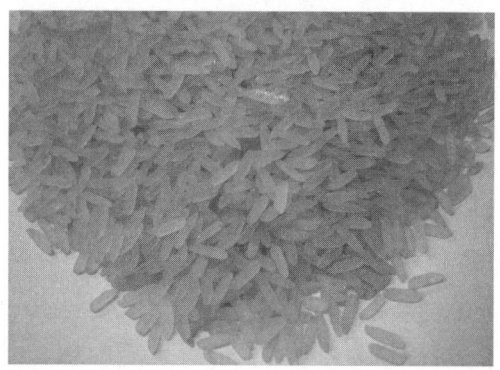

Energy	346 kcal	Moisture	13 gm
Protein	6 gm	Fat	0 gm
Mineral	1 gm	Fibre	0 gm
Carbohydrates	79 gm	Calcium	9 mg
Phosphorous	143 mg	Iron	1 mg

- This is partially boiled in the husk.
- Parboiling drives nutrients, especially thiamine, so 80% nutritionally similar to brown rice.
- Parboiled rice takes less time to cook and is firmer and less sticky.

BROWN RICE

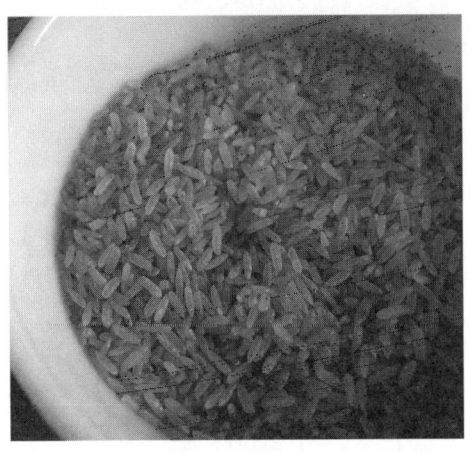

(Amount 1 cup)			
Proteins	15 g	Calories	695
Carbohydrates	146 g	Dietary Fiber	6.6 g
Sugar	1.6 g	Fat	5.3 g
Omega-3 fatty acids	81 mg	Omega-6 fatty acids	1.8 g
Calcium	53 mg	Iron	3.1 mg
Magnesium	272 mg	Phosphorus	567 mg
Potassium	466 mg	Sodium	10 mg
Zinc	3.8 mg	Copper	526 mcg
Manganese	7.1 mg	Selenium	44 mcg
Vitamin E	2.3 mg	Vitamin K	3.6 mcg
Thiamin	773 mcg	Riboflavin	129 mcg
Niacin	8.9 mg	Vitamin B_6	0.97 mg
Folic acid	38 mcg	Pantothenic acid	2.8 mg

- Hulled rice.
- Rice bran oil, in brown rice, contains gamma-oryzanol which lowers LDL cholesterol.
- Beneficial in type 2 diabetes.
- Inhibits growth of malignancy cells, especially pancreatic.
- High in insoluble fiber preventing the formation of gallstones
- Prevents neural tube defect and spina bifida in intrauterine life.
- Helpful in postmenopausal women against high blood pressure, high cholesterol and cardiovascular diseases.
- Useful in high blood pressure and atherosclerosis.
- Rich in selenium which prevents colon malignancy.
- Rich in vitamin E—an antioxidant, helpful against heart disease, atherosclerosis, stroke, asthma and rheumatoid arthritis.

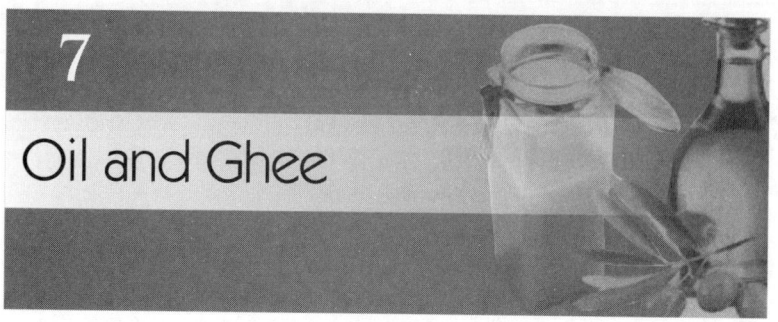

7

Oil and Ghee

CLARIFIED BUTTER GHEE

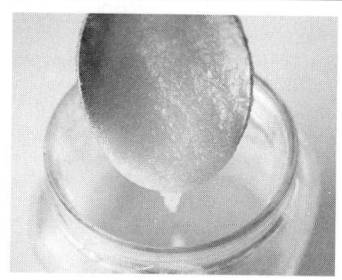

(1 tbsp)

Calories	112	Fat	12.73 g
Saturated fat	7.926 g	Polyunsaturated fat	0.473 g
Monounsaturated fat	3.678 g	Cholesterol	33 mg
Potassium	1 mg	Carbohydrate	0 g
Protein	0.04 g		

VEGETABLE OIL

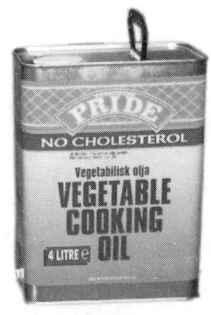

194

(1 tbsp)			
Calories	120	Fat	13.6 g
Saturated fat	1.716 g	Polyunsaturated fat	6.695 g
Monounsaturated fat	4.591 g	Cholesterol	0 mg
Carbohydrateohydrate	0 g	Protein	0 g

CORN OIL

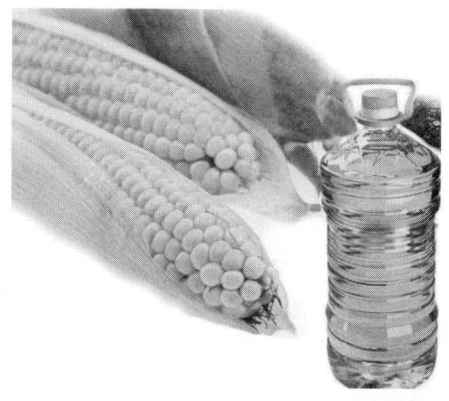

(1 tbsp)			
Calories	124	Fat	14g
Saturated fat	1.302 g	Polyunsaturated fat	6.244 g
Monounsaturated fat	5.852 g		

SUNFLOWER OIL

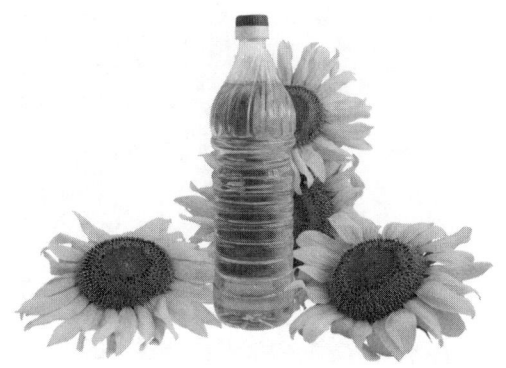

(1 tbsp)			
Calories	120	Fat	13.6 g
Saturated fat	1.402 g	Polyunsaturated fat	8.935 g
Monounsaturated fat	2.652 g	Cholesterol	0 mg
Carbohydrateohydrate	0 g	Protein	0 g

OLIVE OIL

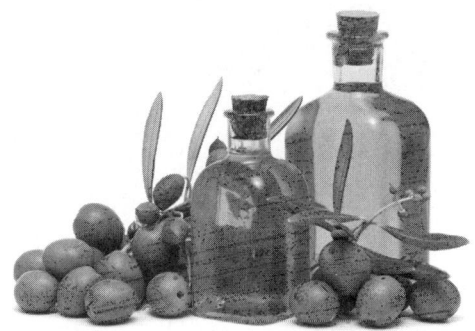

(Per 100 gm)			
Energy	885 kcal	Carbohydrates	0 g
Fat	100 g	Saturated	14 g
Monounsaturated	73 g	Polyunsaturated	11 g
Protein	0 g	Vitamin E	14 mg
Vitamin K	62 µg		

CANOLA OIL

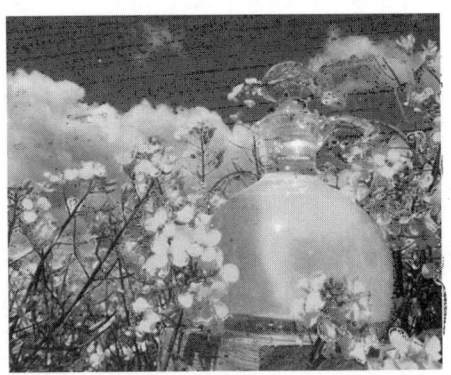

- Healthiest oil.
- Low in saturated fats.
- Contains omega-6 and omega-3-essential fatty acids which are healthiest cooking oils.
- Rich in plant sterols-β-sitosterol and campesterols which reduces the risk of heart disease and also reduces cholesterol.
- Rich in calories which help to lower bad cholesterol and increase good cholesterol.
- Contains antioxidant which prevents from harmful oxygen-free radicals.
- Highest smoke point oil useful for deep frying.

MUSTARD OIL

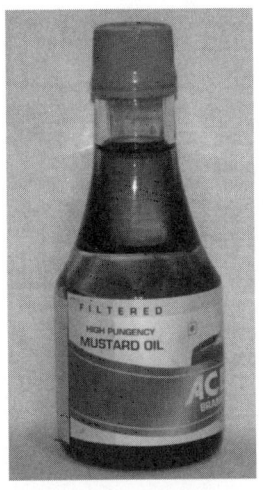

Calories	126	Fat	14
Carbohydrates	0	Fibers	0
Protein	0		

- Protection from coronary heart diseases.
- Has antibacterial and anti-fungal property.
- Reduces hair fall through improved blood circulation.
- Helps in digestion, circulation and excretory system.

- Boosts up immune system.
- Useful in cough and cold.

RICE BRAN OIL

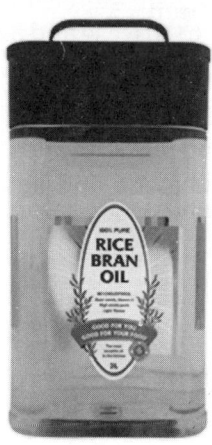

Calories	122.4	Fat	13.6 g
Saturated fat	2.7 g	Monounsaturated fat	5.3 g
Polyunsaturated fat	4.8 g	Cholesterol	0 mg
Sodium	0 mg 0%	Potassium	0 mg
Carbohydrates	0 g	Protein	0 g
Vitamins and minerals			
Vitamin E	4.4 mg	Vitamin K	3.4 g
Iron	0 mg		

- Contains high fractions of tocopherols, tocotrienols and vitamin E.
- Improves blood cholesterol by reducing total plasma cholesterol and triglycerides.
- In relieving hot flashes and other symptoms of menopause.
- Contains antioxidants.
- Has lower amount of mono-unsaturated and poly-unsaturated fats.
- Contains fewer polymers which are richer flavors and easy to clean up.

- Rich in thiamine, niacin and vitamin B_6. Small amount of riboflavin, folic acid and vitamin K.
- Rich in manganese, phosphorus, iron, potassium, zinc and copper.
- Small amount of sodium.
- Reduces cholesterol and cardiovascular disease.
- It modulates pituitary secretion, inhibition of gastric acid secretion, antioxidant action, inhibition of platelet aggregation, lowering of blood pressure and regulation of cholesterol.
- Oil extracted from the germ and inner husk of rice.
- Has high smoke point of 232°C.
- Suitable for high-temperature cooking.

CHEESE

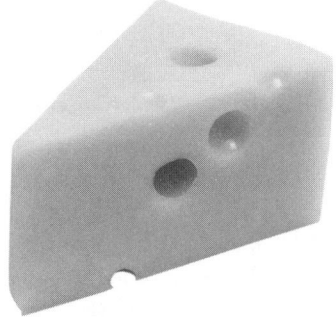

(Per 100 grams)			
Energy	371 calories	Fat	32 g
Saturated fat	18 g	Polyunsaturated fat	1.3 g
Monounsaturated fat	8 g	Trans fat	1.1 g
Cholesterol	100 mg	Sodium	1, 671 mg
Potassium	132 mg	Carbohydrate	3.7 g
Dietary fiber	0 g	Sugar	2.3 g
Protein	18 g		

- Rich in calcium and vitamin B_{12}.
- Useful for children, pregnant women and the elderly.
- Prevents osteoporosis.

- Makes strong teeth.
- Rich in protein, fat and sodium.

BUTTER

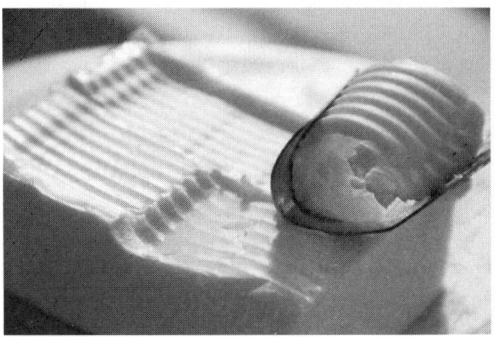

(Per 100 grams)			
Calories	717	Fat	81 g
Saturated fat	51 g	Polyunsaturated fat	3 g
Monounsaturated fat	21 g	Trans fat	3.3 g
Cholesterol	215 mg	Sodium	11 mg
Potassium	24 mg	Carbohydrateohydrate	0.1 g
Dietary fiber	0 g	Sugar	0.1 g
Protein	0.8–1 gm%		

- Rich in vitamin A.
- Gives a feeling of satiety that may decrease cravings and over-eating.
- Contains conjugated linoleic acids which is malignancy protective.
- Good source of iodine necessary for thyroid function.
- Promotes gastro-intestinal health and decreases rates of diarrhea in children.
- Good source of vitamin K_2 which prevents tooth decay and builds strong teeth and bones.
- Rich in antioxidants—vitamins A, E, selenium and protects against heart disease as well as malignancy.

- Good source of dietary cholesterol which is useful for development of the brain in children.
- Consists of short and medium chain fatty acids which have anti-tumor action.

PEANUT OIL

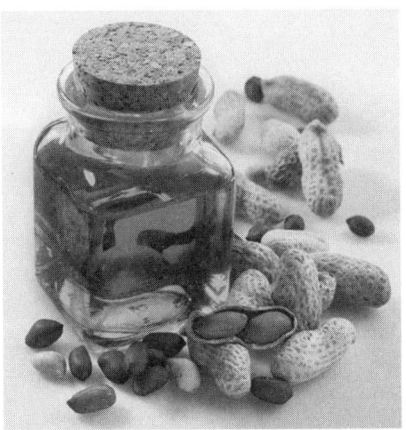

Energy	884 kcal	Carbohydrates	0 g
Protein	0 g	Fat	100 g
Cholesterol	0 mg	Sodium	0 mg
Potassium	0 mg	Calcium	0 mg
Copper	0 mg	Iron	0.03 mg
Magnesium	0 mg	Manganese	0 mg
Phosphorus	0 mg	Selenium	0 µg
Zinc	0.01 mg	Vitamin E	15.69 mg
Vitamin K	0.7 µg		

- Low in saturated fats.
- Free from cholesterol.
- Contains essential fatty acid-omega-6 that lowers LDL cholesterol and increases HDL good cholesterol.
- Contains resveratrol, a polyphenol antioxidant which protects against malignancies, heart disease, degenerative nerve disease and Alzheimer's disease.
- Rich in vitamin E.

- Healthiest cooking oil.
- Good source of plant sterols, especially β-sitosterol. Reduces cholesterol levels.
- High in calories.

SARSON OIL

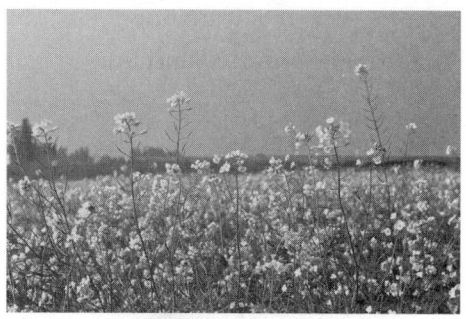

- Strengthens the nervous system.
- Relieves asthma.
- Stabilises blood pressure.
- Alleviates migraine headaches.
- Reduces risk of heart attack and stroke.
- Releases energy from protein and carbohydrate.

PALM OIL

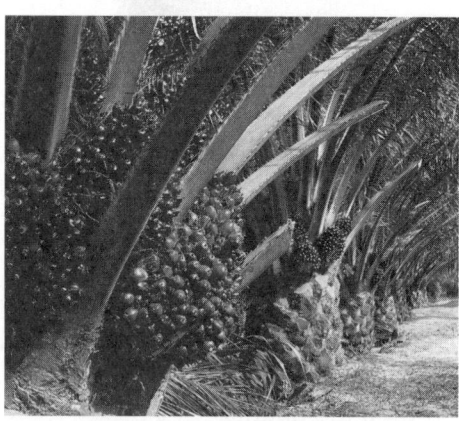

(Per 100 gm)			
Energy	900 kcal	Trans fatty acids	0.5 g
Protein	0.0 g	Fats	100 g
Carbohydrates	0.0 g		

- Rich in vitamin A, carotene, tocopherols and tocotrienol. These act as antioxidant, anticarcinogenic.
- Has perfect balance of saturated and unsaturated fatty acids in India.

REFINED SOYBEAN OIL

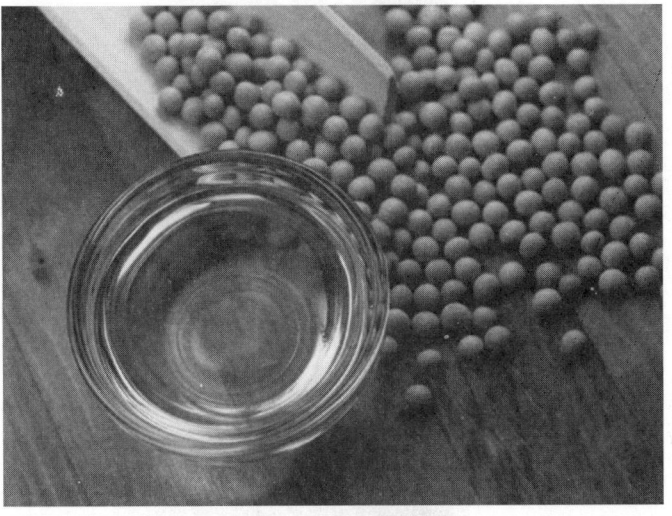

(Per 100 gm)			
Energy	900 kcal	Trans fatty acids	0.0 g
Protein	0.0 g	Carbohydrates	0.0 g
Cholesterol	0.0 g	Fats	100 g

- Cholesterol free.
- Good for heart.
- Contains natural antioxidants.

COTTON SEED OIL

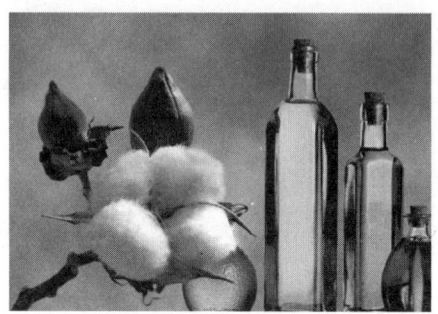

(Per 100 gm)			
Energy	900 kcal	Trans fatty acids	0.0 g
Protein	0.0 g	Carbohydrates	0.0 g
Cholesterol	0.0 g	Fats	100 g

- A healthier edible oil.
- Has medicinal properties.
- Supports chemotherapy in patients of malignancies.
- Has natural antioxidants.

VANASPATI GHEE

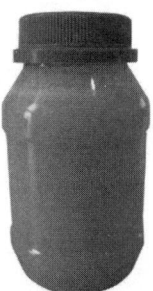

(Per 100 gm)			
Energy	900 cal	Fats	100g
Vitamin A	2500 IU	Carbohydrate	0 gm
Trans fatty acids	0.0 g	Cholesterol	0.0 g
Vitamin D	200 IU	Protein	0.0 gm

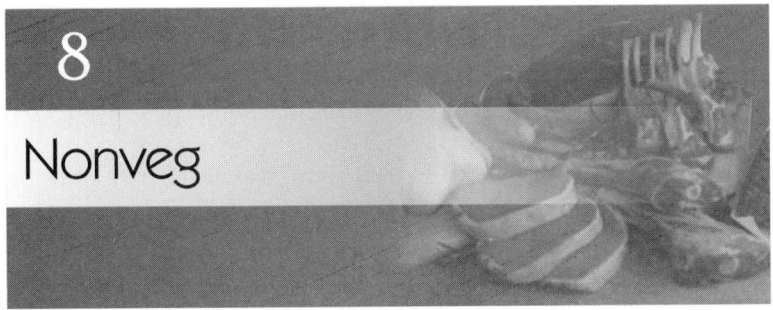

8
Nonveg

CHICKEN EGG

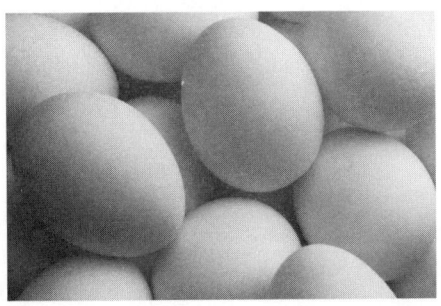

(Per 100 gm)			
Energy	155 calories	Total carbohydrate	1.1 g
Dietary fiber	0 g	Sugar	1.1 g
Protein	13 g	Fat	11 g
Saturated fat	3.3 g	Polyunsaturated fat	1.4 g
Monounsaturated fat	4.1 g	Cholesterol	373 mg
Sodium	124 mg	Potassium	126 mg

- Rich in antibodies-IgY which can treat human rotavirus, *Escherichia coli*, Streptococcus, Pseudomonas, Staphylococcus and Salmonella infections.
- Nutritionally balanced.
- Has high biological.
- Ideal nutritional support for convalescents, tuberculosis or AIDS related infections.

- Egg albumen prevents ulcer formation.
- Rich sources of "sialic acid," which is useful in *Helicobacter pylori* infections causing ulcers, colon malignancy, gastritis and enteritis.
- Contains choline which helps to prevent birth defects, promotes brain and memory development in infants.
- Rich in riboflavin, pantothenic acid, phosphorus, vitamin D, calcium, vitamin E and selenium.
- Helps to maintain a healthy weight.
- Contains G1-globulin lysozyme, the G2 and G3-globulins, ovomacroglobulin, antibody IgY helps to prolong the lives of those with AIDS.
- Contains lumiflavin and lumichrome which restricts the multiplication of malignancy-inducing viruses.

EGG WHITE

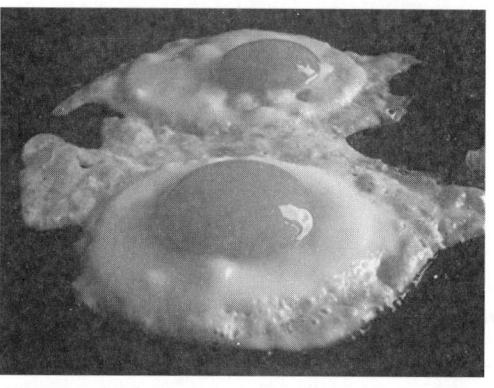

(1 *large*)			
Calories	17	Fat	0.06 g
Cholesterol	0 mg	Sodium	55 mg
Potassium	54 mg	Carbohydrateohydrate	0.24 g
Dietary fiber	0 g	Sugars	0.23 g
Protein	3.6 g		

- Egg contains two liquids—the yolk and the egg white.
- Egg white is the clear liquid that encompasses the yolk and serves as a protector of the embryo.
- Rich in calcium, magnesium, potassium, copper and selenium.
- Rich in riboflavin, pantothenic acid, vitamin B_{12}, folic acid and thiamin.
- Low in calories and fat.
- cholesterol free.
- High in protein useful for malignancy patients undergoing radiotherapy.

CHICKEN EGG, YOLK

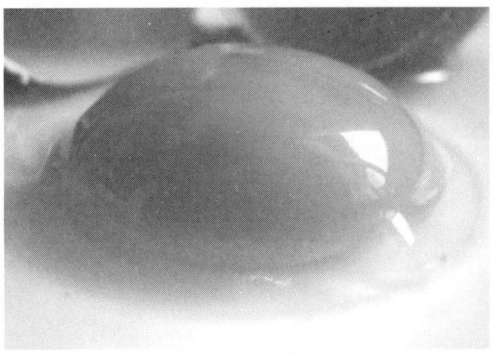

(Per 100 gm)			
Energy	317 kcal	Carbohydrates	3.59 g
Fat	26.54 g	Protein	15.86 g
Calcium	129 mg	Iron	2.73 mg
Magnesium	5 mg	Phosphorus	390 mg
Potassium	109 mg	Zinc	2.30 mg
Cholesterol	1240 mg	Vitamin A	381 µg
Thiamine	0.176 mg	Riboflavin	0.528 mg
Pantothenic acid	2.990 mg	Folic acid	146 µg
Vitamin D	218 IU		

EGG OMELET

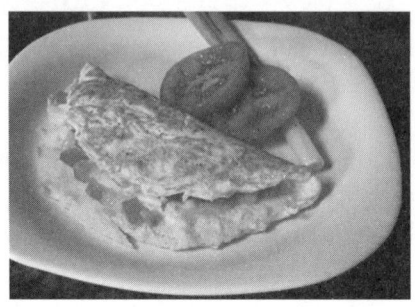

	(*1 large*)		
Calories	93	Fat	7.33 g
Saturated fat	2.053 g	Polyunsaturated fat	1.279 g
Monounsaturated fat	3.044 g	Cholesterol	217 mg
Sodium	98 mg	Potassium	70 mg
Carbohydrate	0.42 g	Dietary fiber	0 g
Sugars	0.4 g	Protein	6.48 g

BOILED EGG

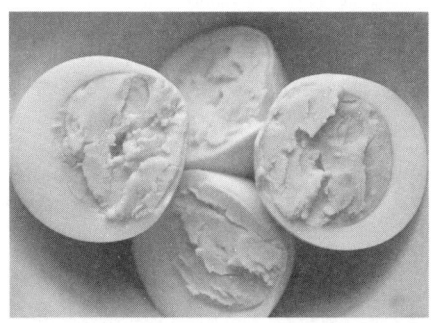

	(*1 large*)		
Calories	77	Fat	5.28 g
Saturated fat	1.627 g	Polyunsaturated fat	0.704 g
Monounsaturated fat	2.03 g	Cholesterol	211 mg
Sodium	139 mg	Potassium	63 mg
Carbohydrate	0.56 g	Dietary fiber	0 g
Sugars	0.56 g	Protein	6.26 g

POACHED EGG

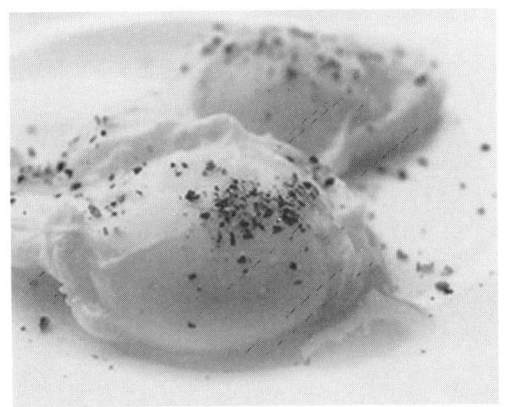

(1 large)			
Calories	73	Fat	4.95 g
Saturated fat	1.543 g	Polyunsaturated fat	0.679 g
Monounsaturated fat	1.897 g	Cholesterol	210 mg
Sodium	147 mg	Potassium	66 mg
Carbohydrate	0.38 g	Dietary fiber	0 g
Sugars	0.38 g	Protein	6.26 g

COOKED EGG

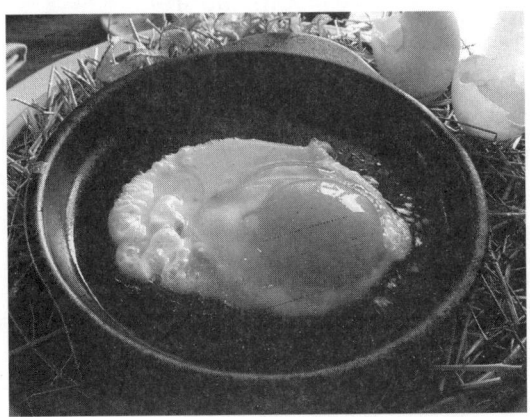

(1 large)			
Calories	84	Fat	6.11 g
Saturated fat	1.807 g	Polyunsaturated fat	0.978 g
Monounsaturated fat	2.427 g	Cholesterol	204 mg
Sodium	179 mg	Potassium	67 mg
Carbohydrateohydrate	0.63 g	Dietary fiber	0 g
Sugars	0.57 g	Protein	6.14 g

DUCK EGGS

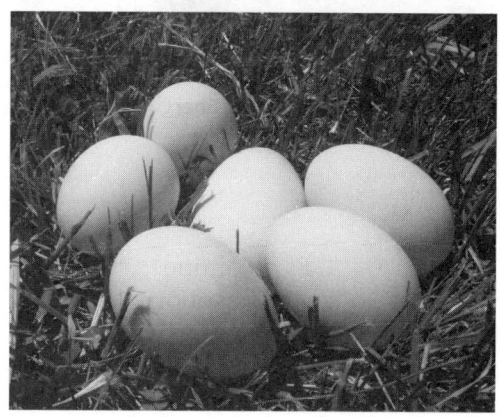

- Energy in 100 gm of egg is 185 kcal.
- Rich in selenium, manganese, zinc, copper, potassium, sodium, phosphorus, calcium and iron.
- Rich in thiamin, niacin, riboflavin, pantothenic acid, folic acid, vitamin B_6, vitamin D, vitamin E, vitamin A, vitamin B_{12} and retinol.
- Anti-malignancy food.
- Have twice the nutritional value of a chicken egg.
- Fat—3.68 gm of saturated fat/100 gm.
- High in cholesterol—884 mg/100 gm.
- Rich in omega-3 fatty acids which improves brain power.
- More vitamin K_2.
- High in protein.

QUAIL EGG

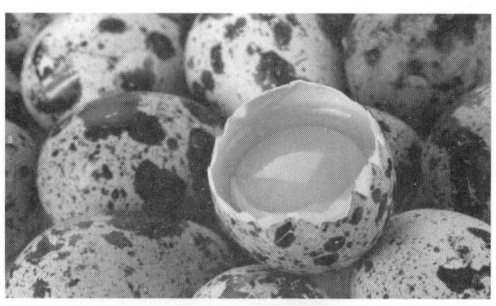

(*One quail egg*)			
Weight	9 gm	Energy	14 calories
Protein	1.2 gm		
No carbohydrates or sugars			
Fat	1 gm	Cholesterol	76 mg

- Rich in vitamins A, B_{12}, B_6, thiamine, riboflavin, niacin, beta-carotene and lutein. Rich in phosphorus, potassium, selenium and calcium, and smaller amount of iron, manganese, copper and zinc.

CHICKEN

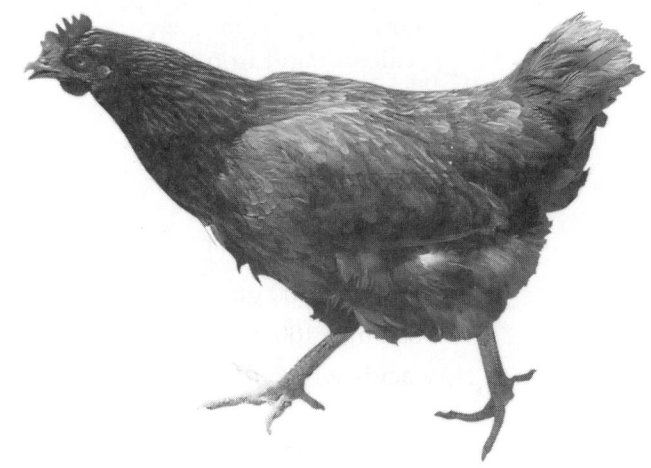

(Per 4.00 oz-wt)			
Calories	223.40 g	Protein	33.79 g
Fat	8.82 g	Saturated fat	2.48 g
Mono fat	3.44 g	Poly fat	1.88 g
Calcium	15.88 mg	Copper	0.06 mg
Iron	1.21 mg	Magnesium	30.62 mg
Manganese	0.02 mg	Phosphorus	242.68 mg
Potassium	277.83 mg	Selenium	28.01 mg
Sodium	80.51 mg	Zinc	1.16 mg
Vitamin A	105.46 IU	Niacin B_3	14.41 mg
Folic acid	4.54 mcg		

- Rich in vitamin B_6 which boosts up immune system.
- Rich in niacin or vitamin B_3.
- Maintains normal functioning of thyroid gland.
- Contains phosphorus, potassium, zinc.

CHICKEN-TANDOOR

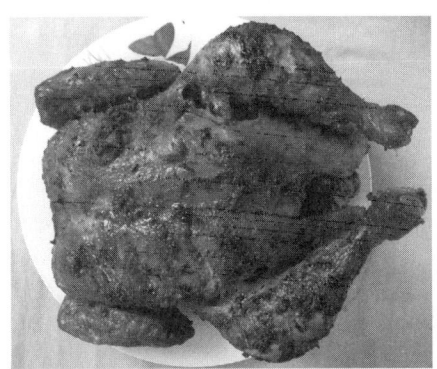

(100 gm)			
Energy	197 calories	Protein	29.80 gm
Fat	7.78 gm	Potassium	245 mg
Phosphorus	214 mg	Calcium	14 mg
Magnesium	27 mg	Iron	1.07 mg
Sodium	71 mg	Manganese	0.018 mg
Zinc	1.02 mg	Vitamin B_6	0.56 mg
Folic acid	4 mcg	Vitamin B_{12}	0.32 mcg
Vitamin A	93 IU		

CHICKEN SOUP

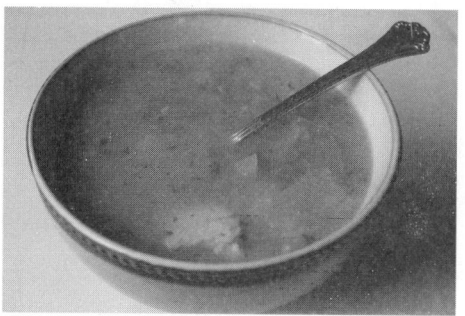

(1 cup)			
Calories	75	Fat	2.46 g
Saturated fat	0.651 g	Polyunsaturated fat	0.554 g
Monounsaturated fat	1.109 g	Cholesterol	7 mg
Sodium	1106 mg	Potassium	55 mg
Carbohydrateohydrate	9.35 g	Dietary fiber	0.7 g
Sugars	0.27 g	Protein	4.05 g

FISH

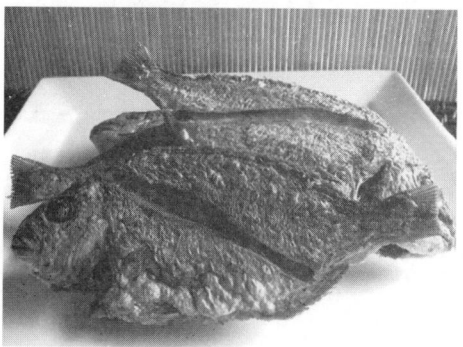

- Highly nutritious food.
- Excellent protein.
- Low in calories.
- Rich in omega-3 fatty acids which is good for the heart.
- Perfect for weight loss plan.

White fish:			
Energy	321 kJ	Protein	17 g
Fat	7 g	Water	8 g
Calcium	16 mg	Iron	0.3 mg
Vitamin A	0	Thiamine	0.07 mg
Oily fish:			
Energy	970 kJ	Protein	17 g
Fat	18 g	Water	64 g
Calcium	33 mg	Iron	8 mg
Vitamin A	45	Thiamine	0 mg

- No carbs.
- Rich in vitamins A and D.

MUTTON

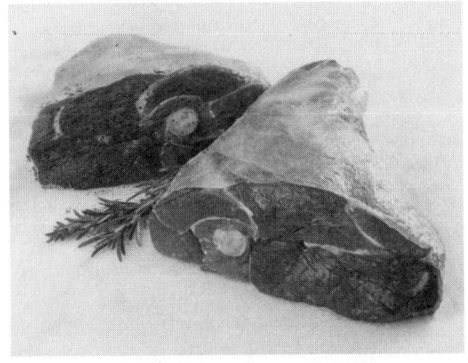

(Goat meat per 100 gm)			
Energy	456	Protein	20.60
Fat	2.31	Calcium	13
Iron	2.83	Phosphorus	180
Potassium	385	Sodium	82
Zinc	4.00	Copper	0.256
Manganese	0.038	Selenium	8.8
Niacin	3.750	Vitamin B$_{12}$	1.13
Fatty acids, total saturated	0.710	Cholesterol	57

- Contains essential amino acids which help to maintain the cardiovascular health.
- Boosts up immune system.
- Rich in phosphorous which maintains bones and teeth growth.
- Low in sodium and high in potassium.
- Rich in thiamin, riboflavin, niacin and cobalamin.
- Rich in iron, zinc, phosphorous, potassium, selenium and omega fatty acids.
- Maintains the blood sugar levels.
- Contains unsaturated fat which lowers the bad cholesterol.
- Rich in protein and energy.
- Prevents warts.

BEEF

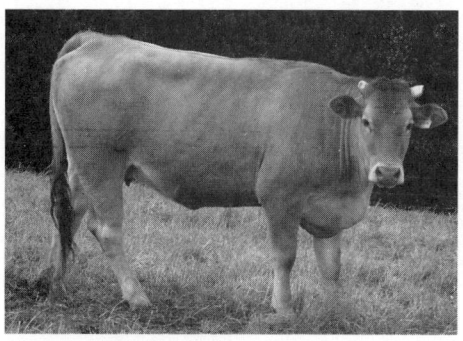

(Per 4.00 oz-wt)			
Protein	32.04 g	Cholesterol	95.25 mg
Calories	240.41 kJ	Fat	11.45 g
Thiamin B_1	0.15 mg	Riboflavin B_2	0.35 mg
Niacin B_3	4.44 mg	Niacin	10.41 mg
Vitamin B_6	0.49 mg	Vitamin B_{12}	2.92 mcg
Vitamin D mcg	0.35 mcg	Vitamin E	0.23 mg
Folic acid	7.93 mcg	Pantothenic acid	0.43 mg
Calcium	7.93 mg	Copper	0.20mg
Iron	4.05 mg	Magnesium	34.03 mg
Manganese	0.01 mg	Phosphorus	269.89 mg
Molybdenum	3.85 mcg	Potassium	475.15 mg
Selenium	27.67 mcg	Sodium	71.44 mg
Zinc	6.33 mg		

- Domestic cattle (like cows).
- Beef is the third most widely consumed meat in the world.
- High nutritional value.
- Rich in zinc, selenium, phosphorus, iron and B vitamins.
- There is strong evidence that red meat are causes of bowel malignancy.
- Contains high levels of undesirable saturated fat so there is high incidence of coronary heart disease and diabetes mellitus.

PORK

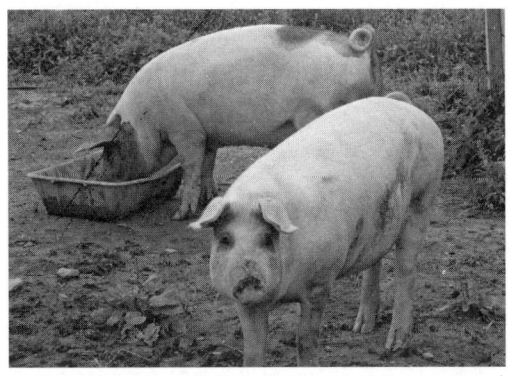

(Per 100 g)			
Energy	242 kcal	Carbohydrates	0.00 g
Sugars	0.00 g	Dietary fibre	0.0 g
Fat	13.92 g	Protein	27.32 g
Calcium	19 mg	Iron	0.87 mg
Magnesium	28 mg	Phosphorus	246 mg
Potassium	423 mg	Sodium	62 mg
Zinc	2.39 mg	Vitamin B_6	0.464 mg
Vitamin B_{12}	0.70 µg	Vitamin C	0.6 mg
Vitamin D	53 IU		

- Carriers of diseases like pork tapeworm , trichinosis, various helminthes, such as roundworms, pinworms, hookworms and hepatitis E.

CRAB

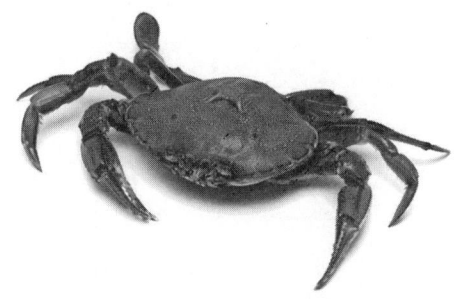

(Amount 85 gm)			
Protein	17 gm	Calories	87
Fat	1.5 gm	Saturated fat	0.2 gm
Monounsaturated fat	0.2 gm	Polyunsaturated fat	0.6 gm
Sodium	237 mg	Potassium	235 mg

- Types—blue crabs, dungeness crabs, king crabs, stone crab and red crab.
- Low in calories and fat.
- Healthy for heart.
- Rich source of lean protein for athletes, sportsperson and body builders and also for diabetics.
- Good source of omega-3 fatty acids which lowers triglycerides and blood pressure.
- Boost up immunity.
- High amount of mercury.
- Good source of chromium, selenium, vitamin B_{12}, zinc and copper.

LOBSTER

- Seafood.
- 100 g of lobsters have 90 calories.
- Rich in sodium, potassium and phosphorus, calcium, magnesium, iron, zinc, copper, manganese and selenium.
- Small amount of vitamins K, B_{12} and folic acid.

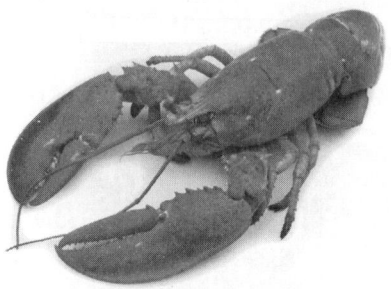

- Rich in omega-3 fatty acids which keep away the heart problems. They are good for eyes, healthy bones and generate energy in the body.

FROG LEGS

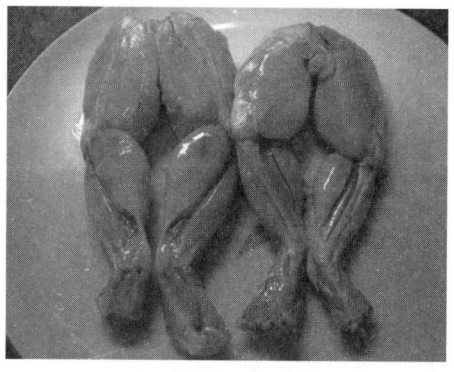

(Per 100 gm)			
Energy	73 kcal	Protein	16.4 g
Fat	0.3 g	Calcium	18 mg
Cholesterol	50 mg	Copper	0.25 mg
Folic acid	15 mcg	Iron	1.5 mg
Magnesium	20 mg	Niacin	1.2 mg
Phosphorus	147 mg	Potassium	285 mg
Selenium	14.1 mcg	Sodium	58 mg
Thiamin	0.14 mg	Vitamin A	50 IU
Vitamin B_{12}	0.4 mcg	Vitamin B_6	0.12 mg
Vitamin E	1 mg	Vitamin K	0.1 mcg
Zinc	1 mg		

SHEEP, MUTTON

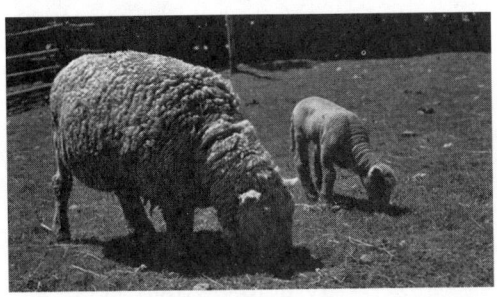

(Per 100 gm)			
Energy	236 kcal	Protein	17.9 g
Carbohydrate	0.1 g	Sodium	55 mg
Potassium	220 mg	Calcium	5 mg
Magnesium	16 mg	Phosphorus	120 mg
Iron	2.3 mg	Zinc	2.9 mg
Copper	0.08 mg	Manganese	0.01 mg
Vitamin A	12 µg	Vitamin E	0.6 mg
Vitamin K	6 µg	Vitamin B_1	0.06 mg
Vitamin B_2	0.22 mg	Vitamin B_3	3.8 mg
Vitamin B_6	0.13 mg	Vitamin B_{12}	2 µg
Vitamin B_9	1 µg	Vitamin B_5	0.72 mg
Vitamin C	1 mg	Cholesterol	77 mg

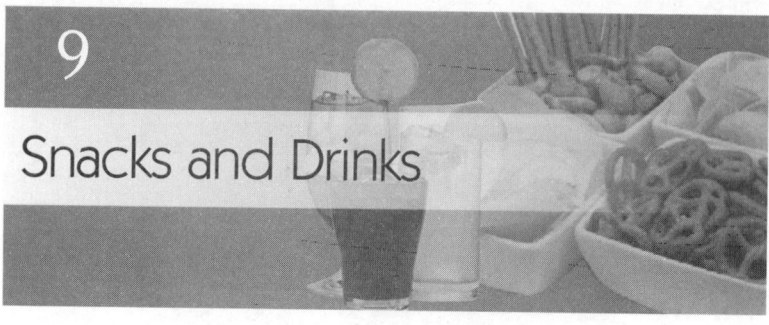

9
Snacks and Drinks

POHAY

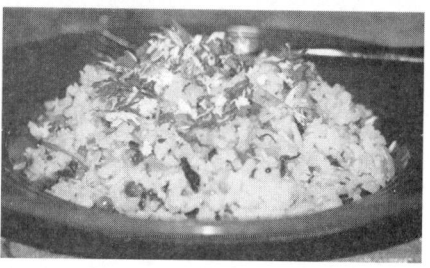

Carbohydrate 68.9 gm	Proteins 6.8 gm	Fats 6 gm

Pohay is made of flattened, processed rice, roasted with chilies, onions, mustard and cumin seeds and curry leaves. It is a high carbohydrate, low fat, quick meal that can be made in minutes. Pohay is easily available in most tea shops and other restaurants.

UPAMA

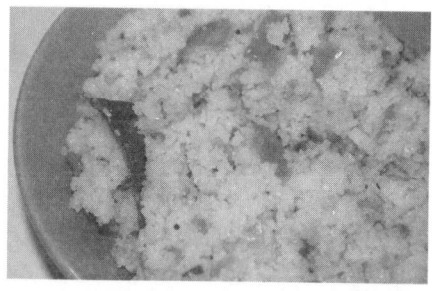

Quantity 116.6 gm			
Carbohydrates	44.9 gm	Proteins	8.1 gm
Fats	3.7 gm	Total calories	248 cal
Fiber	3.2 gm	Sodium	0.39 gm

SAMOSA

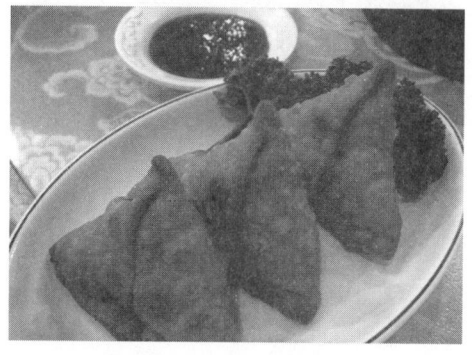

Carbohydrates	48.1 gm	Proteins	6.3 gm
Fats	17.3 gm	Total calories	369 cal

SABUDANA KHICHADI

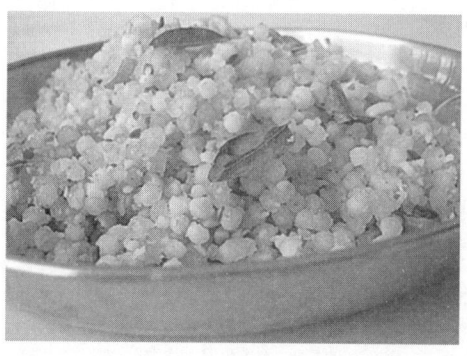

Quantity 127.7 gm			
Carbohydrates	20.5 gm	Proteins	2.7 gm
Fats	9.0 gm	Total calories	169 cal
Quantity	127.7 gm		

METHI PAROTHA

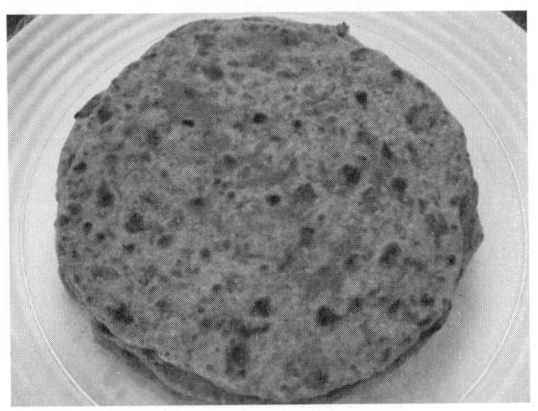

Quantity 70 gm			
Carbohydrates	36.3 gm	Proteins	6.8 gm
Fats	1.4 gm	Total calories	180 cal
Fiber	4.2 gm	Sodium	0.14 gm

CORNFLAKES

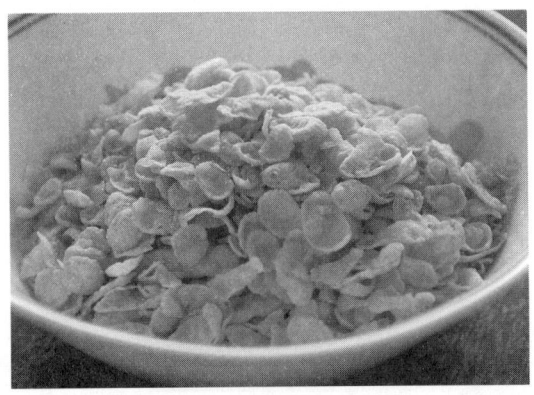

Quantity (gm) 30 in 50 ml milk			
Carbohydrates	28.5 gm	Proteins	3.4 gm
Fats	0.2 gm	Total calories	124 cal

IDLI

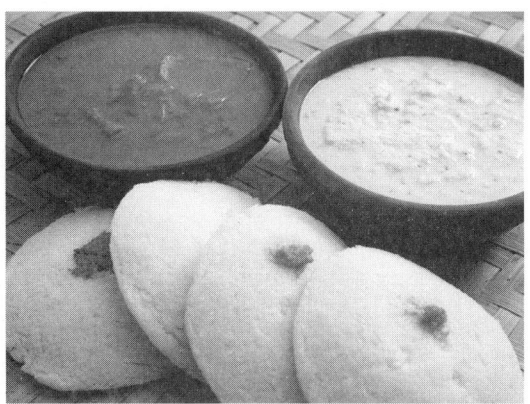

	Quantity 1 pc.		
Carbohydrates	15 gm	Proteins	1.2 gm
Fats	0.2 gm	Total calories	69 cal.

BOILED EGGS

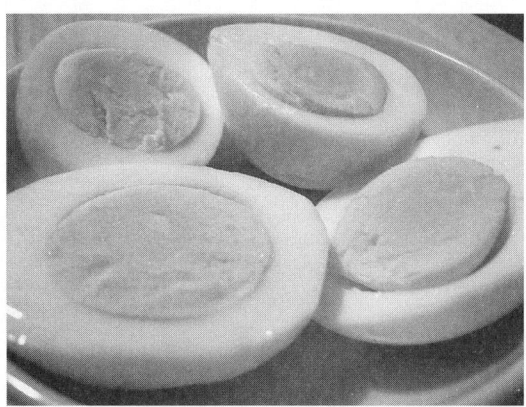

	Quantity (gm) 83 gm 1 pc.		
Carbohydrates	0.6 gm	Proteins	9.8 gm
Fats	5 gm	Total calories	91 cal.

OMELET

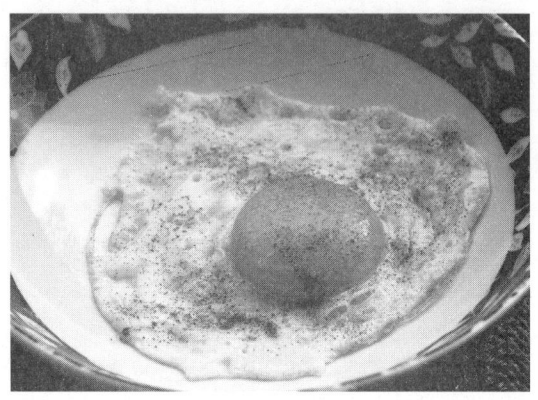

Quantity 185.8 gm			
Carbohydrates	2.7 gm	Proteins	17.8 gm
Fats	24.5 gm	Total calories	303 cal.

BHURJEE

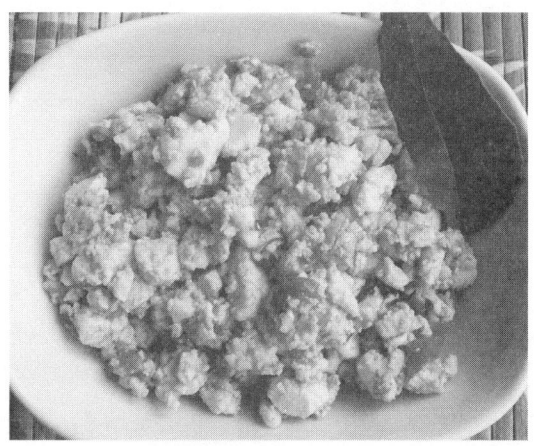

Quantity 102.9 gm			
Carbohydrates	0.8 gm	Proteins	12.6 gm
Fats	11.8 gm		

DOSAS

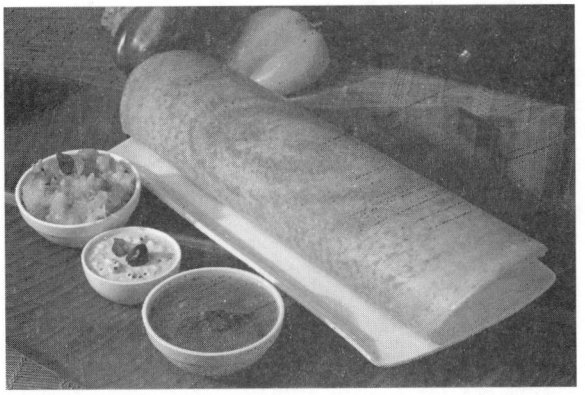

Calories	145 kcal	Proteins	2.8 g
Fats	5.2 g		

UTTAPAM

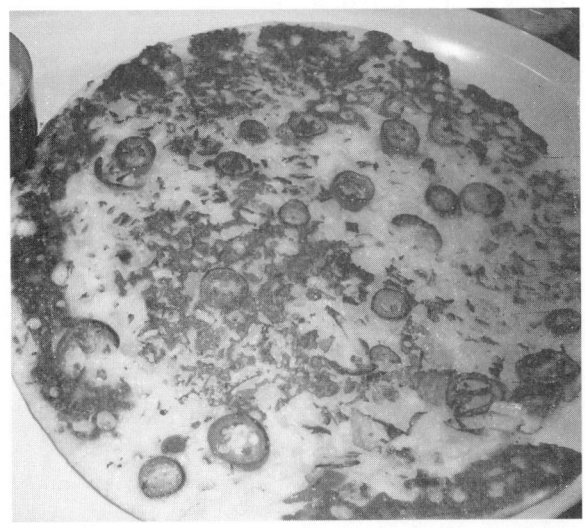

		170 kcal	
Proteins	3 g	Fat	7 g

PAV BHAJI

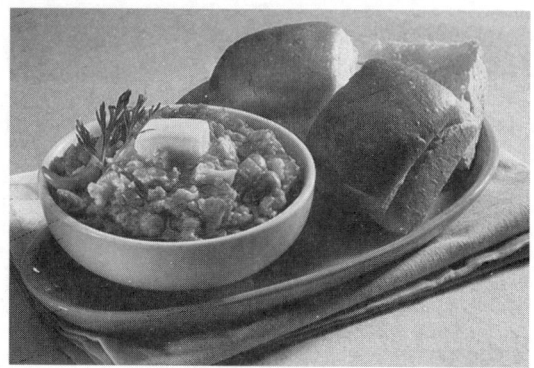

Calories	160.0	Fat	9.0 g
Saturated fat	2.0 g	Polyunsaturated fat	0.0 g
Monounsaturated fat	0.0 g	Cholesterol	5.0 mg
Sodium	640.0 mg	Potassium	0.0 mg
Carbohydrateohydrate	18.0 g	Dietary fiber	3.0 g
Sugars	0.0 g	Protein	3.0 g

OATMEAL

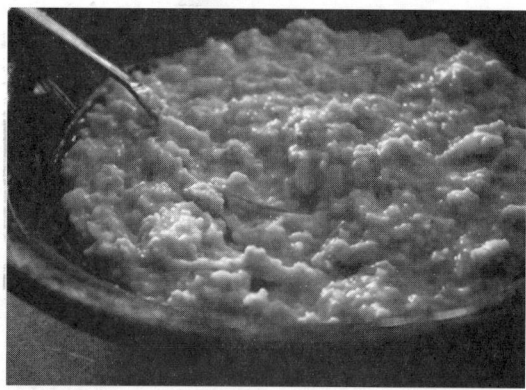

1 cup of cooked			
Calories	145 kcal	Fat	2.39 g
Carbs	25.37 g	Protein	6.06 g

TOASTED BREAD

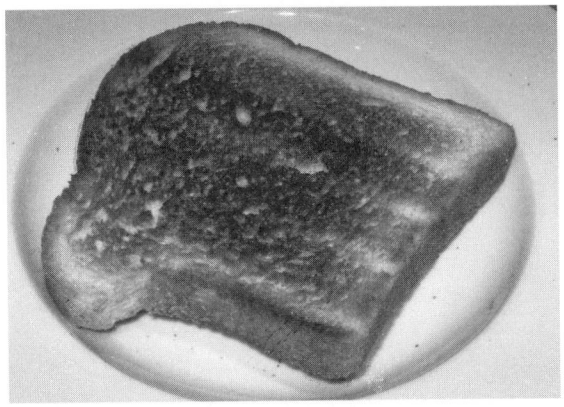

Per 1 regular slice			
Calories	70 kcal	Fat	0.96 g
Carbs	13.06 g	Protein	2.16 g

BREAD

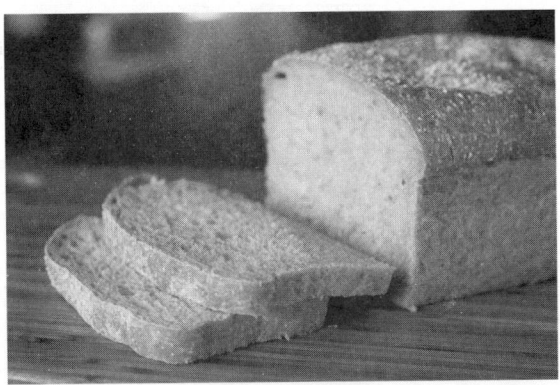

2 pieces			
Calories	190	Fat	5 gm
Sodium	110 mg	Carbohydrateohydrate	11 gm
Protein	3 gm		

BLACK RASPBERRY JAM

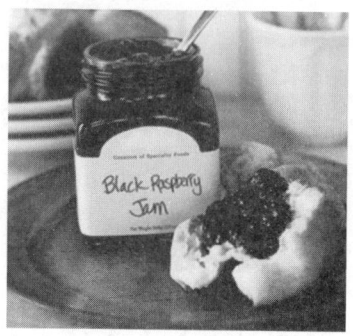

1 tbsp

Calories	50.0	Fat	0.0 g
Saturated fat	0.0 g	Polyunsaturated fat	0.0 g
Monounsaturated fat	0.0 g	Cholesterol	0.0 mg
Sodium	0.0 mg	Potassium	0.0 mg
Carbohydrateohydrate	13.0 g		

STRAWBERRY JAM

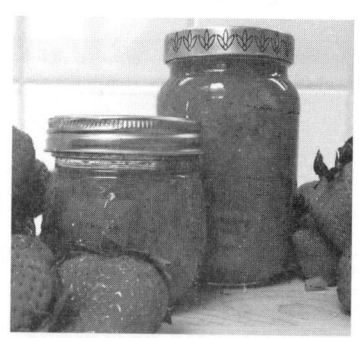

15 gm serving

Calories	40.0	Fat	0.0 g
Sodium	2.0 mg	Potassium	0.0 mg
Carbohydrateohydrate	10.0 g	Dietary fiber	0.0 g
Sugars	10.0 g	Protein	0.0 g
Vitamin A	0.0 %	Vitamin B	120.0 %

PINEAPPLE JAM

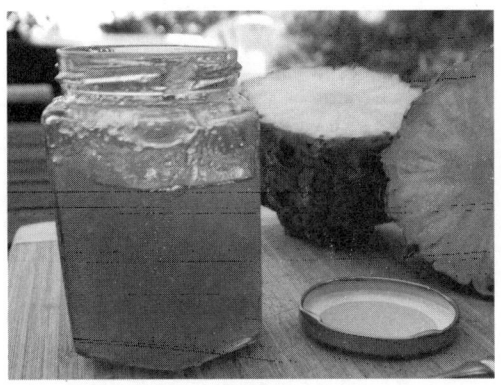

	Per 1 tbsp		
Calories	50.0	Carbohydrate	13.0 g
Sugars	12.0 g	Protein	0.0 g
Vitamin B	120.0 %		

VADA PAV

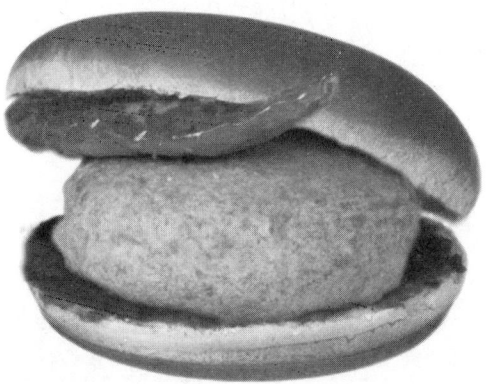

	Serving size 1		
Calories	290 kcal	Fat	20 g
Carbs	25 g	Protein	5 g

POTATO CHIPS

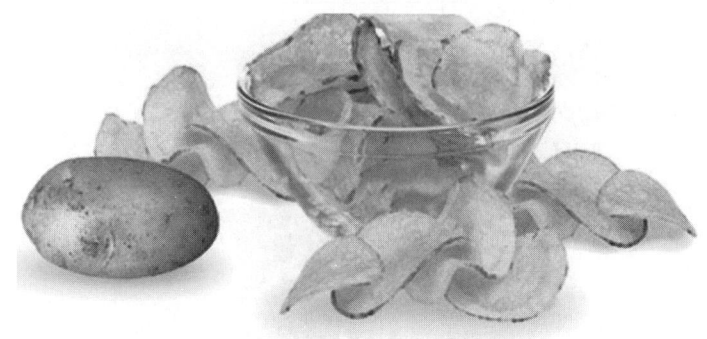

Energy	554 kcal	Protein	7.0 g
Carbohydrate	52.7 g	Sugars	1.3 g
Fat	35 g		

CUBE OF SUGAR

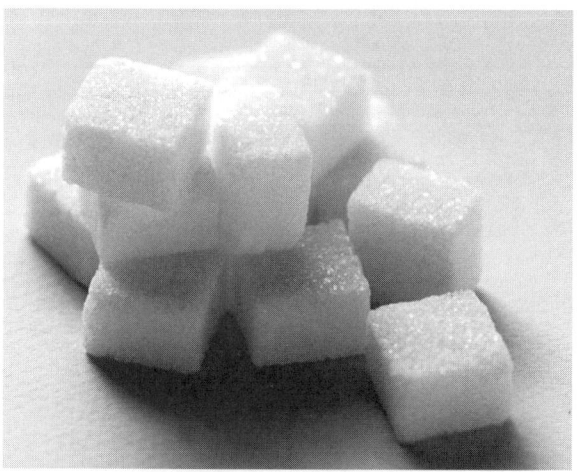

- Cube of sugar weighs 4 g.
- 4 calories per gram.
- 1 sugar cube—15 to 16 calories.
- Relatively low in calories.

MASALA MAGGI

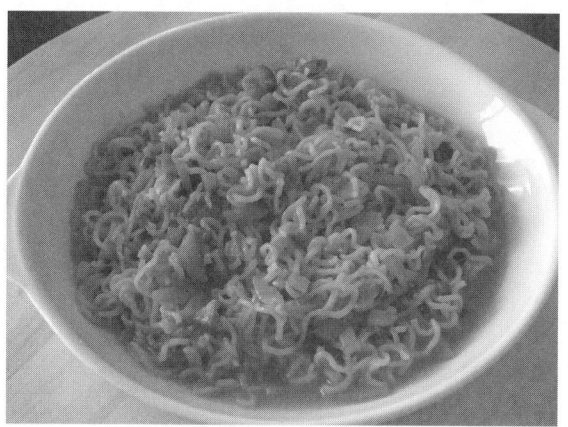

Protein	9.2 g	Carbohydrate	58.9 g
Sugars	1.2	Fat	14.4 g
Trans fat	Not mentioned	Calcium	150 mg
Potassium	365 mg		

BURGERS

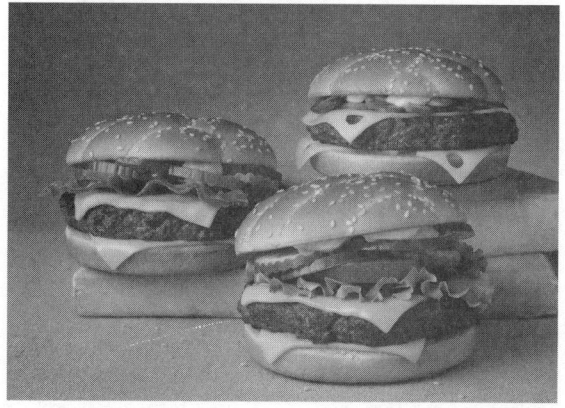

Salt (g/day)	1.8	Carbohydrate (g/day)	43.4
Fat (g/day)	10.5	Trans fat (g/day)	0.4

FRIES

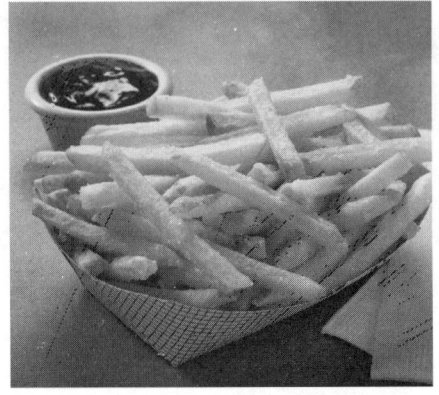

| Salt (g/day) | 0.4 | Carbohydrate (g/day) | 46.5 |
| Fat (g/day) | 19.9 | Trans fat (g/day) | 1.6 |

PAPAD

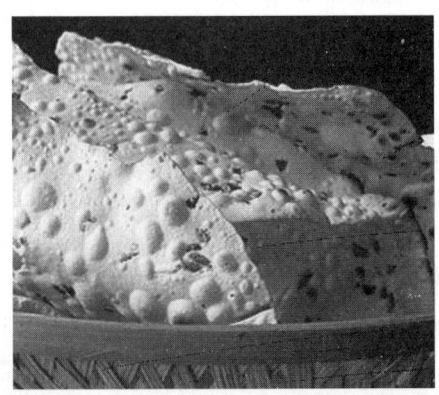

	Per 100 gm		
Calories	371	Fat	3.3 g
Saturated fat	1.1 g	Cholesterol	4 mg
Sodium	1745 mg	Carbohydrate	60 g
Dietary fiber	19 g	Sugar	0 g
Protein	26 g		

KISSAN—MIXED FRUIT JAM

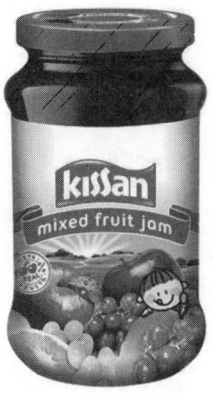

20 gm			
Calories	65	Sodium	10 mg
Carbohydrates	16 g	Sugars	16 g

MIXED FRUIT JELLY

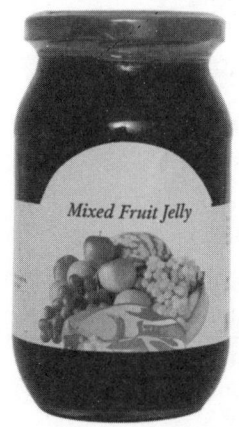

Per 1 tbsp			
Calories	50.0	Carbohydrateohydrate	13.0 g
Dietary Fiber	0.0 g	Sugars	12.0 g
Vitamin B	120.0%	Vitamin B	60.0%

TOMATO SAUCE

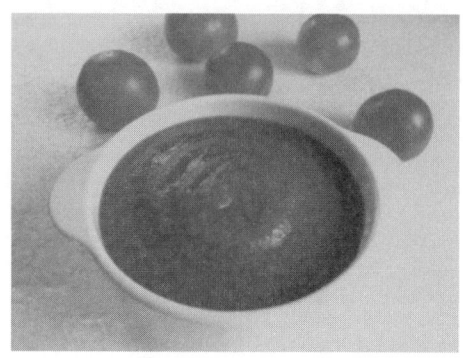

	100 gm		
Calories	29	Fat	0.2 g
Sodium	11 mg	Potassium	331 mg
Carbohydrateohydrate	7 g	Dietary fiber	1.5 g
Sugar	4.2 g	Protein	1.3 g

CHINESE GARLIC SAUCE

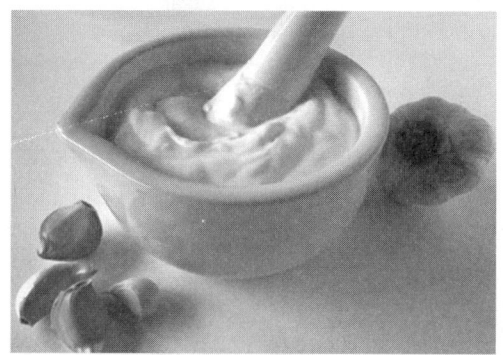

	Per 1 cup		
Calories	668.0	Fat	57.0 g
Saturated fat	10.0 g	Vitamin B	120.0%
Vitamin B	60.0%	Protein	10.0 g

SOY SAUCE

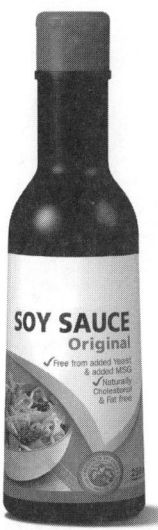

Per 1 tbsp			
Energy	8 kcal	Protein	1 g
Carbohydrate	1.22 g	Sugar	0.27 g
Fat	0.01 g	Saturated fat	0.001 g
Monounsaturated fat	0.001 g	Polyunsaturated fat	0.003 g
Cholesterol	0 mg	Fibre	0.1 g
Sodium	902 mg	Potassium	35 mg

PIZZA

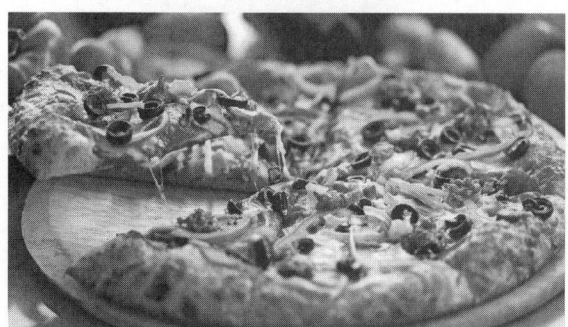

Per 100 gm			
Calories	266	Fat	10 g
Saturated fat	4.5 g	Polyunsaturated fat	1.7 g
Monounsaturated fat	2.6 g	Trans fat	0.2 g
Cholesterol	17 mg	Sodium	598 mg
Potassium	172 mg	Carbohydrate	33 g
Dietary fiber	2.3 g	Sugar	3.6 g
Protein	11 g		

- High fat cheeses.
- High intake contributes to obesity—a risk factor for malignancy.

HAMBURGER

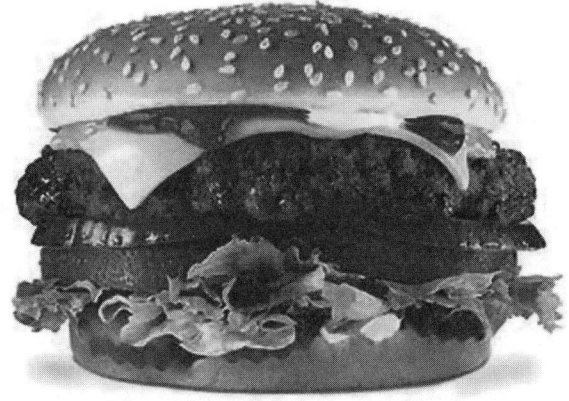

Per 100 gm			
Calories	295	Fat	14 g
Saturated fat	5 g	Trans fat	0.8 g
Cholesterol	47 mg	Sodium	414 mg
Potassium	226 mg	Carbohydrate	24 g
Dietary fiber	0.9 g	Sugar	4.2 g
Protein	17 g		

PASTA

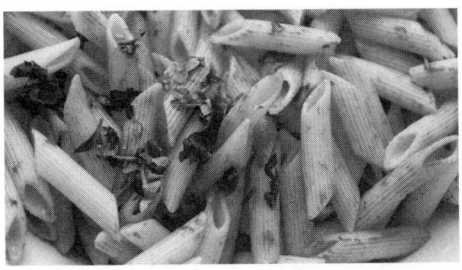

(Per 100 gm)			
Calories	158	Fat	0.9 g
Saturated fat	0.2 g	Polyunsaturated fat	0.3 g
Monounsaturated fat	0.1 g	Sodium	1 mg
Potassium	44 mg	Carbohydrate	31 g
Dietary fiber	1.8 g	Sugar	0.6 g
Protein	6 g		

- Low in calories.
- Rich in magnesium, iron, calcium, potassium, zinc, selenium and manganese
- Releases energy, slowly providing energy for a longer time.
- Small amount of sodium.
- No cholesterol.
- Rich in iron and vitamin B.
- Low glycemic index.

SPAGHETTI

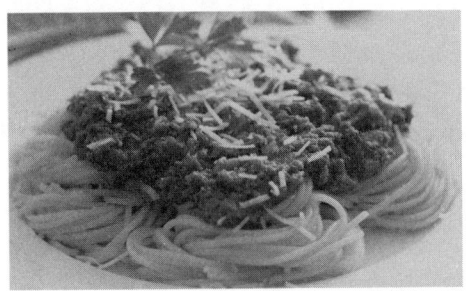

(Per 100 gm)			
Calories	158	Fat	0.9 g
Saturated fat	0.2 g	Polyunsaturated fat	0.3 g
Monounsaturated fat	0.1 g	Sodium	1 mg
Potassium	44 mg	Carbohydrate	31 g
Dietary fiber	1.8 g	Sugar	0.6 g
Protein	6 g		

- Long, thin, cylindrical pasta of Italian and Sicilian origin. Spaghetti is made of semolina or flour and water.

SHEER KHURMA

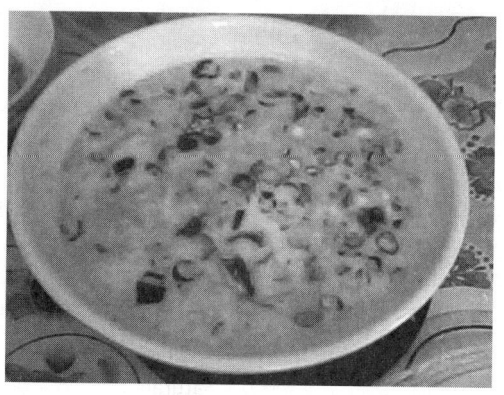

Quantity 1 pc.			
Calories	232	Fat	5 g
Carbs	51 g	Protein	3 g

- Prepared by Muslims on Eid ul-Fitr, traditional Muslim festive breakfast and a dessert for celebrations.
- Sheer is milk and khurma is dates.
- Special dish is served on the morning of Eid day in the family after the Eid prayer as breakfast and throughout the day to all the visiting guests.

Ingredients:
- Whole milk 1 liter

- 5 to 6 dried dates
- 1/2 cup vermicelli
- 2 to 3 tsp butter or vegetable ghee
- 10 to 12 chopped almonds (thin sliced)
- 10 to 12 chopped cashews (thin sliced)
- 10 to 12 raisins
- 4 to 5 small cardamom or 1 tsp cardamom powder
- 2 cup sugar (as per taste).

SHRIKHAND

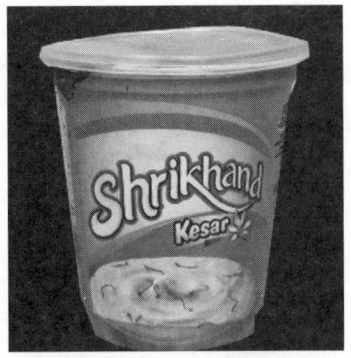

Calories	130	Sodium	15 mg
Fat	4 g	Saturated	2 g
Carbohydrates	23 g	Dietary fiber	0 g
Sugars	21 g	Protein	4 g
Cholesterol	10 mg		

AMUL SHRIKHAND

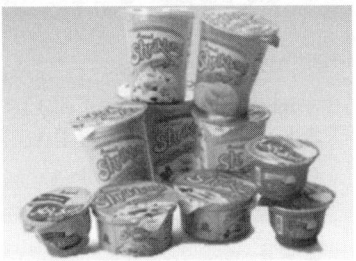

(Per 100 g)			
Energy	279 kcal	Fat	7 g
Saturated fat	4 g	Cholesterol	0.020 mg
Sodium	30 mg	Carbohydrateohydrate	46 g
Protein	8 g		

KESAR SHRIKHAND

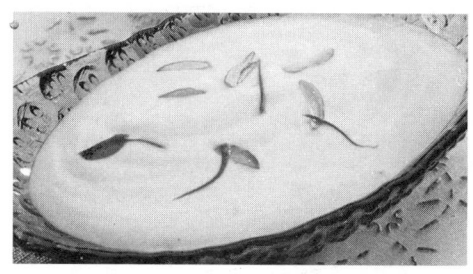

(½ serving)			
Calories	281	Fat	5 g
Carbs	4 g	Protein	1 g

AMRAKHAND

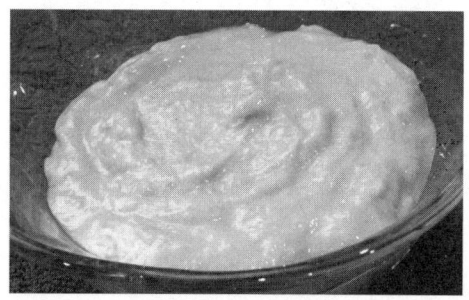

(Per 100 gm)			
Energy	0.80 kcal	Fat	6.80 g
Carbohydrates	50.62 g	Protein	9.28 g
Cholesterol	9.00 g	Vitamin A	6.20 g
Vitamin C	3.30 g	Iron	0.033 g
Calcium	134.53 g	Sodium	18 g

AMUL MANGO SHRIKHAND

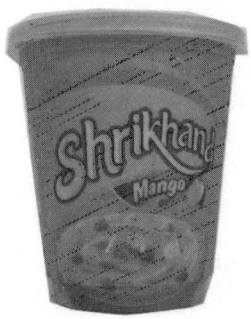

(Per 50 g)			
Calories	130	Fat	3.5 g
Saturated fat	2 gm	Cholesterol	10 mg
Carbohydrate	23 gm	Protein	3 gm
Calcium	2%		

BREAD, FRENCH OR VIENNA

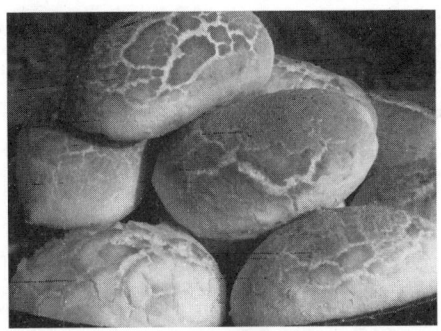

(100 gm)			
Calories	289	Fat	1.8 g
Saturated fat	0.5 g	Polyunsaturated fat	0.8 g
Monounsaturated fat	0.3 g	Sodium	513 mg
Potassium	128 mg	Carbohydrate	56 g
Dietary fiber	2.4 g	Sugar	2.6 g
Protein	12 g		

GREEN TEA

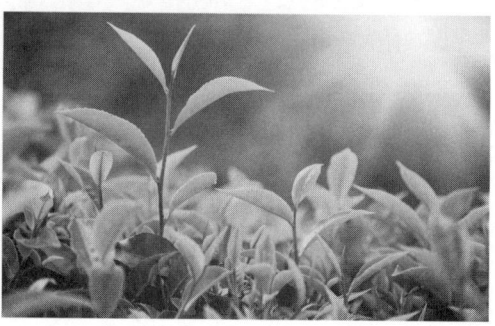

Calories	2	Fat	0 g
Carbs	0.47 g	Protein	0 g

- Made from the leaves of *Camellia sinensis* that have undergone minimal oxidation during processing.
- Rich in branched-chain amino acids which is useful in *chronic liver diseases* and *liver malignancy.*
- Helps in growth of beneficial intestinal microflora.
- Lower blood low-density lipoprotein and total cholesterol levels, reduces the risk of coronary artery disease.
- Reduces body fat.
- Rich in polyphenols and flavonoids alkaloids like caffeine and theobromine, carbohydrate and stannins.
- Rich in fluoride and aluminium.
- Contains epigallocatechin gallate—powerful antioxidants.
- Very rich in catechin which has anti-malignancy properties.
- Acts as anti-obesity, antidiabetic, and anti-inflammatory.
- Prevents dental caries.
- Controls blood pressure, prevents coronary heart diseases and diabetes.
- Prevents the rise of homocysteine.
- Contains caffeine which increases alertness.

- Prevents Parkinson's disease and also baldness by stimulating the hair follicles.
- Acts as natural antiseptic.
- Has anti-aging property.
- Decreases bad cholesterol by 2–5%.
- Rich in L-theanine amino acid which has calming effect on both body and mind.
- Have germicidal and germistatic property.

BLACK TEA

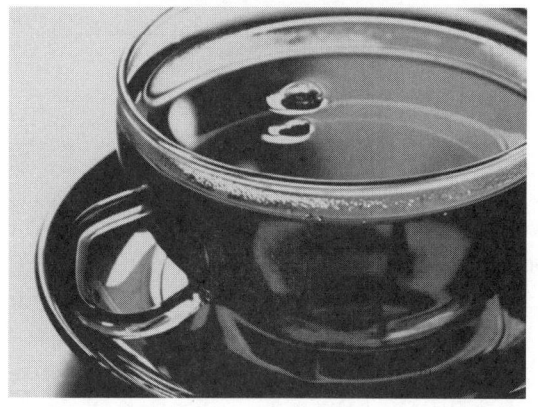

Calories	17	Fat	0.84 g
Carbs	1.51 g	Protein	0.95 g

- Tea that is more oxidized than green and white teas.
- Plain black tea without sweeteners or additives contains negligible quantities of calories, protein, sodium, and fat.
- Reverses endothelial vasomotor dysfunction in coronary artery disease. But addition of milk prevents vascular protective effects of tea.
- Contains theaflavin-3-gallate reduce bad cholesterol level in body.

WHITE TEA

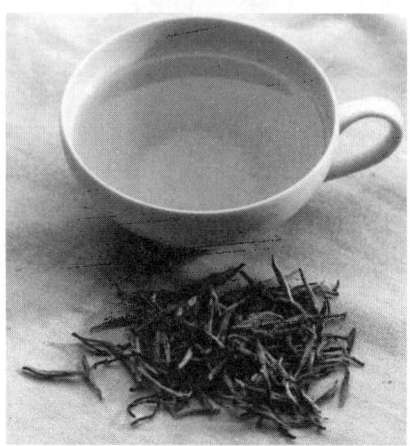

Calorie	2	Fat	0 g
Protein	0 g	Carbohydrate	1 g

- Lightly oxidized tea.
- Derived from *Camellia sinensis*.
- Contains most antioxidants which protects against certain types of malignancy.
- Contains catechins which reduces bad cholesterol, decreases blood pressure and decreases the risk of cardiovascular disease.
- Reduces the incidence of Staphylococcus and Streptococcus infections, pneumonia and fungus growth.
- Boosts up immune systems.
- High anti-inflammatory, antioxidant and anti-collagenase.
- Prevents rheumatoid arthritis, malignancies and heart disease.
- Effective at fighting the bacteria especially in gum disease, plaque and halitosis.

Side effects of tea:
- Contains oxalates which leads to kidney stones.
- Contains fluoride which can cause osteofluorosis and fractures.

- Contains methylxanthine-caffeine which causes a rise in blood pressure, a heart stroke and glaucoma.
- Caffeine a diuretic and also disturbs sleep patterns and causes insomnia.
- In pregnancy can lead to miscarriages.
- Lactating women should avoid tea—baby will have bowel irritability.
- Prolonged or excessive consumption of black tea leads to ovarian malignancy, uterine malignancy, diabetes, hypertension, irritable bowel syndrome and anemia.
- Tea should not be taken within one hour before and after meal, it cannot allow the iron of the meal to absorb in the body.
- Adding milk to tea negates all good effects of tea because casein present in the milk binds with the beneficial epigallocatechin-3-gallate (EGCG) and prevents it from exercising a relaxing effect on arteries.

PARLE G

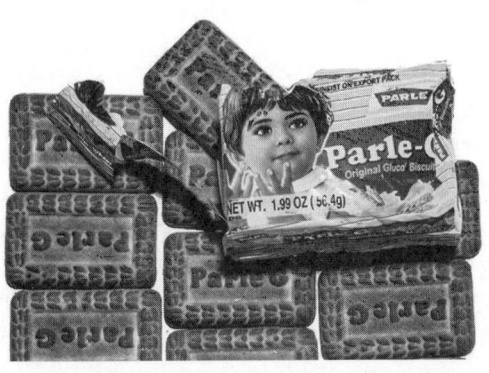

Per 5 pieces			
Total calories	110 kcal	Fat	3.6 g
Saturated fat	1.5 g	Trans fat	0 g
Cholesterol	0 mg	Sodium	75 mg
Carbohydrateohydrate	21 g	Dietary fiber	0 g
Sugars	7 g	Protein	1.8 g
Iron	2%		

MARIE

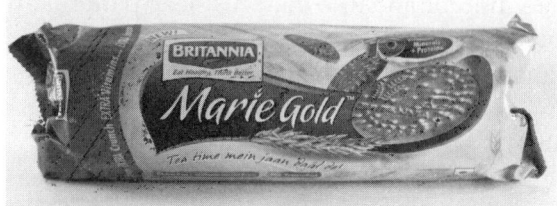

Per 100 gm			
Calories	440 kcal	Sodium	135 mg
Fat	10.9 g	Potassium	0 mg
Saturated	5 g	Carbohydrates	25 g
Polyunsaturated	0 g	Dietary fiber	0 g
Monounsaturated	4 g	Sugars	22 g
Protein	8 g	Cholesterol	0 mg
Vitamin B_1	0.12 mg	Calcium	90 mg
Vitamin B_2	0.14 mg		

TIGER

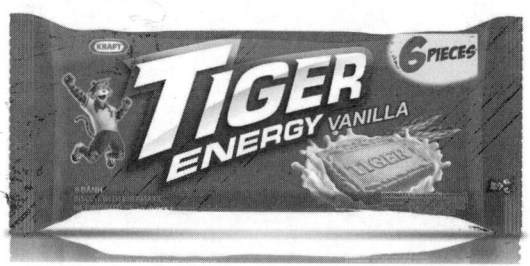

Per 100 gm			
Calories	468 kcal	Fat	20 g
Potassium	0 mg	Saturated	8.5 g
Carbohydrates	66 g	Polyunsaturated	2 g
Dietary fiber	0 g	Monounsaturated	8.2 g
Sugars	24 g	Trans	0 g
Protein	6 g	Cholesterol	0 mg

KRACKJACK

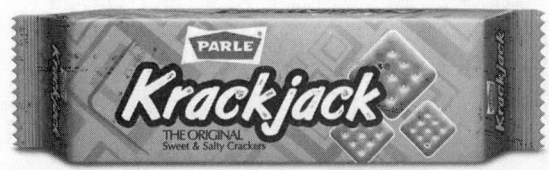

	Per 100 gm		
Calories	475 kcal	Sodium	0 mg
Fat	19 g	Potassium	0 mg
Saturated	9 g	Carbohydrates	69 g
Polyunsaturated	1.5 g	Dietary fiber	0 g
Monounsaturated	0 g	Sugars	20 g
Trans	0 g	Protein	2 g
Cholesterol	0 mg		

GOOD DAY

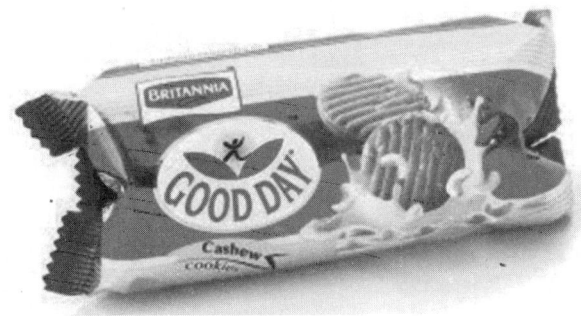

	Per 100 gm		
Calories	491 kcal	Sodium	0 mg
Fat	22 g	Potassium	0 mg
Saturated	11 g	Carbohydrates	66 g
Polyunsaturated	1.9 g	Dietary fiber	2 g
Monounsaturated	8 g	Sugars	24 g
Trans	0 g	Protein	22 g
Cholesterol	13.8 mg		

HIDE AND SEEK COOKIES

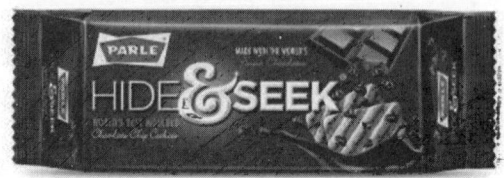

Per 100 gm			
Calories	482 kcal	Sodium	0 mg
Fat	18 g	Potassium	0 mg
Saturated	0 g	Carbohydrates	74 g
Polyunsaturated	0 g	Dietary fiber	0 g
Monounsaturated	0 g	Sugars	32 g
Trans	0 g	Protein	6 g

CREAM BISCUITS

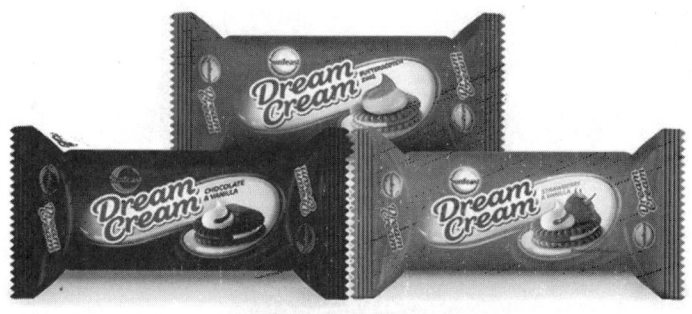

Per 100 gm			
Calories	470 kcal	Fat	19 g
Saturated fat	10 g	Polyunsaturated fat	2 g
Monounsaturated fat	7 g	Cholesterol	0 mg
Potassium	1 mg	Carbohydrateohydrate	69 g
Dietary fiber	0 g	Sugars	39 g
Protein	5.8 g		

LITTLE HEARTS

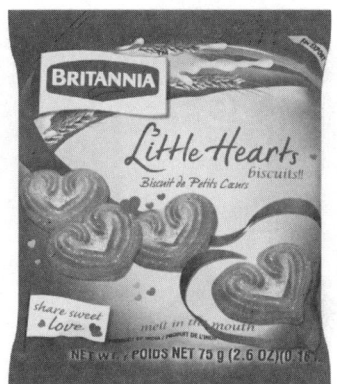

Per 100 gm			
Calories	474 kcal	Sodium	105 mg
Fat	18 g	Potassium	0 mg
Saturated	10 g	Carbohydrates	71 g
Polyunsaturated	1 g	Dietary fiber	0 g
Monounsaturated	6 g	Sugars	26 g
Trans	0 g	Protein	7 g
Cholesterol	0 mg		

SUNFEAST DARK FANTASY—CHOCO FILLS

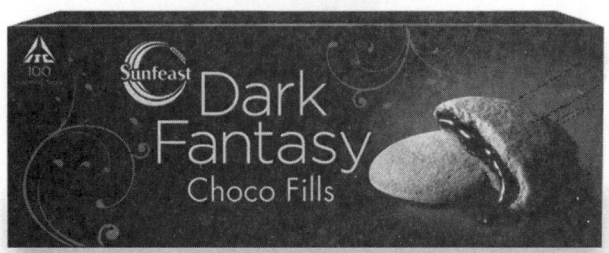

Per 100 gm			
Carbohydrate	63.99 gm	Protein	5.8 gm
Fat	25.1 gm	Energy	505 kcal

BRITANNIA TREAT BISCUITS (100 GM)

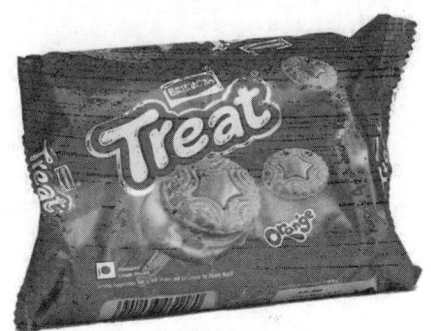

	Per 100 gm		
Carbohydrate	67.5 gm	Protein	5.5 gm
Fat	18.5 gm	Saturated fatty acid	7 gm
Monounsaturated fatty acid	7 gm	Polyunsaturated fatty acid	1 gm
Trans fatty acid	0	Energy	445 cal

FROOTI

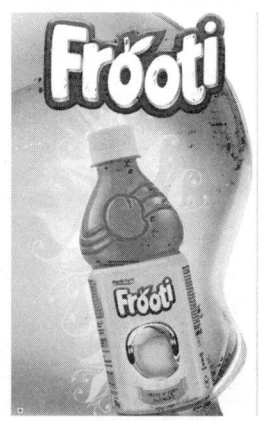

	Per 100 ml		
Calories	61	Fat	0.2 gm
Carbohydrateohydrate	16 gm	Sugars	13 gm
Protein	Less than 1 gm		

COCONUT WATER

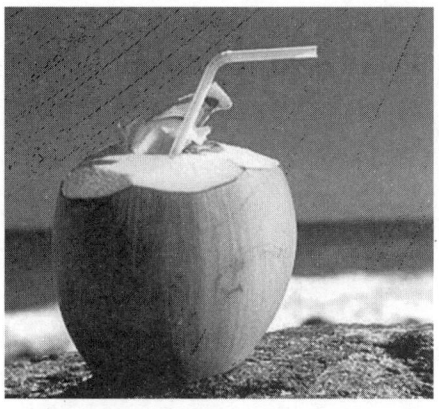

1 cup 240 g			
Calories	46	Fat	0.5 g
Saturated fat	0.4 g	Cholesterol	0 mg 0%
Sodium	252 mg 11%	Carbohydrates	8.9 g 3%
Dietary fiber	2.6 g 11%	Sugars	6.3 g
Protein	1.7 g		

- Very refreshing drink.
- Contains simple sugar, electrolytes, and minerals to replenish hydration levels within the body.
- Contains cytokinins-kinetin and trans-zeatin have anti-ageing, anti-carcinogenic, and anti-thrombotic properties.
- Contains naturally occurring bioactive enzymes—acid phosphatase, catalase, dehydrogenase, diastase, peroxidase, RNA-polymerases, etc. These help in the digestion and metabolism.
- Rich in calcium, iron, manganese, magnesium and zinc.
- Good source of riboflavin, niacin, thiamin, pyridoxine, and folic acid.
- Very good amount of potassium.
- Small amount of vitamin.
- Used in diarrhea to replace the fluid loss from the gastro-intestinal tract and reduce the need for intravenous therapy.

- Osmolarity of tender coconut water is slightly greater than that of WHO recommended ORS.
- Very low in sodium and chlorides.
- Rich in sugars and amino acids.

COCONUT MILK

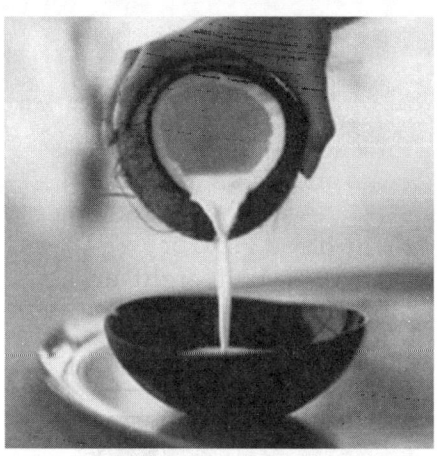

- Coconut milk is obtained by extracting juice by pressing the grated coconut's white kernel or by passing hot water or milk through grated coconut, which extracts the oil and aromatic compounds.
- Contains fat 17%.

COCONUT OIL

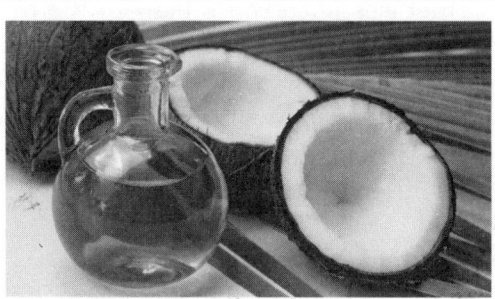

Per 100 gm			
Energy	862 kcal	Carbohydrates	0 g
Protein	0 g	Fat	100 g
Total saturated	86.5 g	Short chain fatty acids	0 g
Medium chain fatty acids	58.7 g	Vitamin E	0.20 mg
Vitamin K	0.5 µg	Iron	0.04 mg
Phyto-nutrients		Phytosterols	86 mg

- High in saturated fats.
- Gives early satiety and increase blood HDL/total cholesterol levels.
- Contains lauric acid and other MCTs absorb passively into the bloodstream and thus save energy and bring early sense of satiety.
- MCTs help raise blood HDL or
- Help to control body weight and decreased risk of atherosclerosis.

SUGARCANE

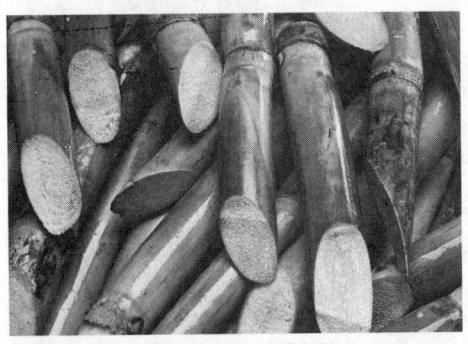

1 oz			
Calories	111.43	Proteins	0.20 g
Water	0.19 g	Fat	0.09 g
Carbohydrates	27.40 g	Sugar	25.71 g
Calcium	32.57 mg	Iron	0.57 mg
Magnesium	2.49 mg	Phosphorus	0.01 mg
Potassium	162.86 mg	Copper	0.09 mg
Manganese	0.09 mg	Riboflavin	0.16 mg
Niacin	0.20 mg	Pantothenic acid	0.09 mg

- Contains no simple sugars, hence can be taken by diabetics.
- Stabilizes blood glucose levels.
- Helps in losing weight.
- Source of instant energy in summers.
- Good for diabetic patients due to its low glycemic index.
- Preventing and treating sore throat, cold and flu.
- Prevents prostate and breast malignancy.
- Helps in the treatment of jaundice for speedy recovery.
- Helpful in urinary tract infections, sexually transmitted diseases, kidney stones and prostatitis.
- Helpful in acidity, genorrhoea, enlarged prostate, cystitis and nephritis.

COFFEE

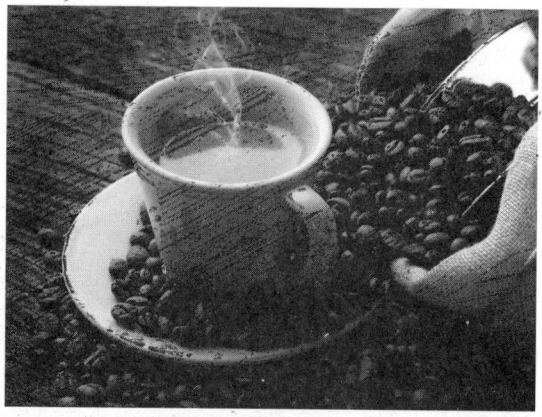

Per 100 gm			
Calories	0	Fat	0 g
Cholesterol	0 mg	Sodium	2 mg
Potassium	49 mg	Carbohydrate	0 g
Dietary fiber	0 g	Sugar	0 g
Protein	0.1 g	Caffeine	40 mg

- Roasted seeds shrub of coffee.
- Reduces the risk of Alzheimer's disease, dementia, Parkinson's disease, heart disease, diabetes mellitus type 2, non-alcoholic fatty liver disease, cirrhosis, and gout.
- Aggravate pre-existing conditions such as gastroesophageal reflux disease, migraines, arrhythmias and sleep disturbances.
- May have depression, anxiety, low vigor, or fatigue.
- Caffeine alleviates headaches.
- Roasted coffee—antioxidant.
- Contains caffeine which acts as an acute antidepressant.
- Contains diterpenes-kahweol and cafestol, which gives increased risk of coronary heart disease.
- Lead to iron deficiency anemia by interfering with iron absorption.

ICED COFFEE

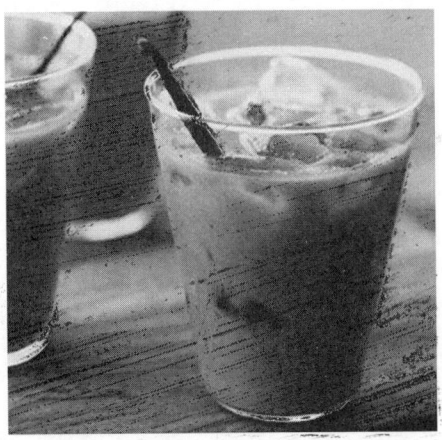

1 coffee cup (6 fl oz)			
Calories	4	Fat	0.01 g
Sodium	4 mg	Potassium	57 mg
Carbohydrate	0.67 g	Protein	0.19 g

FALOODA

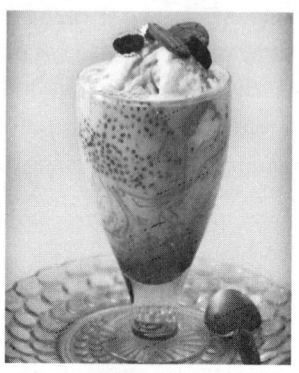

Serving size: 1 (135 g)			
Calories	217.7	Fat	12.6 g
Cholesterol	14.9 mg	Sodium	176.7 mg
Carbohydrate	21.2 g	Dietary fiber	1.1 g
Sugars	0.0	Protein	5.8 g 11%

LIMCA

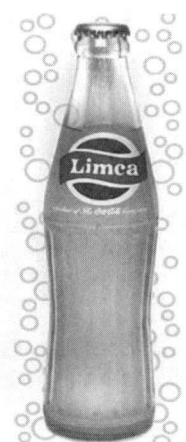

Per 100 ml			
Energy	48 kcal	Carbohydrate	12 gm
Sugar	12 gm	Protein	0 gm
Fat	0 gm		

COCA COLA

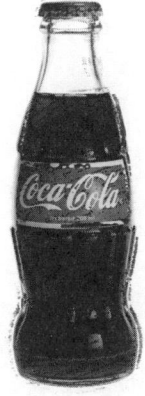

Per 100 ml			
Energy	48 kcal	Carbohydrate	12 gm
Sugar	12 gm	Protein	0 gm
Fat	0 gm		

DIET COKE

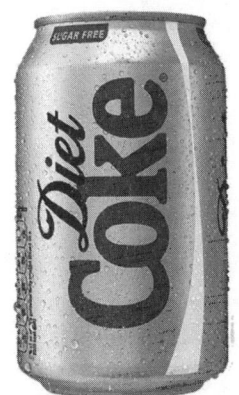

Per 100 ml			
Energy	0.2 kcal	Carbohydrate	0 gm
Sugar	0 gm	Protein	0 gm
Fat	0 gm		

THUMS UP

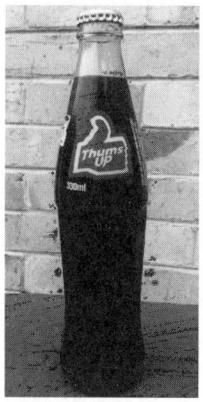

Per 100 ml			
Energy	40 kcal	Carbohydrate	10 gm
Sugar	10 gm	Protein	0 gm
Fat	0 gm		

SPRITE

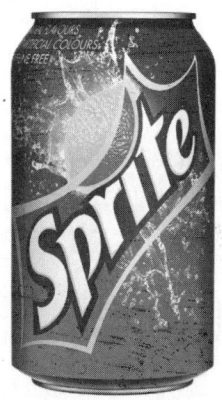

Per 100 ml			
Energy	48 kcal	Carbohydrate	12 gm
Sugar	12 gm	Protein	0 gm
Fat	0 gm		

FANTA

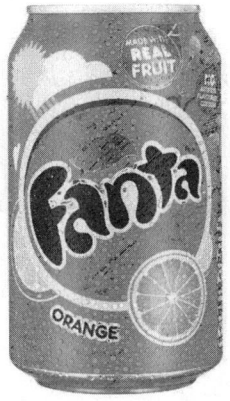

Per 100 ml			
Energy	52 kcal	Carbohydrate	13 gm
Sugar	13 gm	Protein	0 gm
Fat	0 gm		

MAAZA

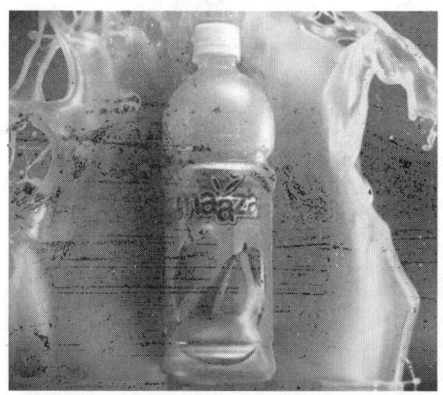

Per 100 ml			
Energy	53 kcal	Carbohydrate	13 gm
Sugar	13 gm	Protein	0 gm
Fat	0 gm		

GLUCON-D

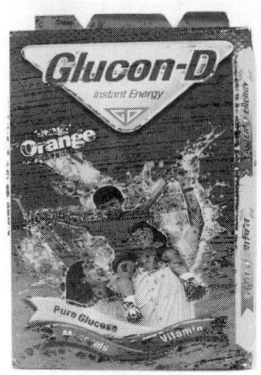

Calories	33	Fat	0 g
Carbohydrates	8 g	Cholesterol	0 mg

BOOST

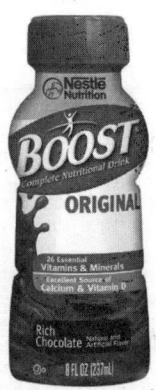

8 oz (227 g)

Calories	240	Fat	4.1 g 6%
Saturated fat	0.5 g	Cholesterol	5 mg
Sodium	130 mg	Carbohydrates	40.0 g
Dietary fiber	0.0 g	Sugars	27.0 g
Protein	10.0 g	Vitamin A	25%
Vitamin C	100%	Calcium	30%
Iron	20%		

BOURNVITA

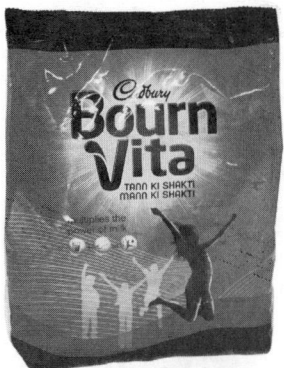

Serving size 1 mug (227 g)			
Calories	173	Fat	6.8 g
Carbohydrates	15.9 g	Dietary fiber	0.0 g
Protein	6.8 g	Energy	173 kcal
Total lipid (fat)	6.81 g		

COMPLAN CHOCOLATE

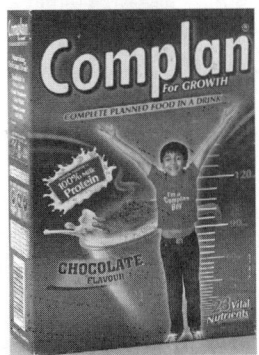

55 gm			
Calories	247	Sodium	105 mg
Fat	9 g	Potassium	0 mg
Saturated	5 g	Carbohydrates	29 g
Polyunsaturated	0 g	Dietary fiber	0 g
Monounsaturated	0 g	Sugars	19 g
Protein	12 g		

HORLICKS

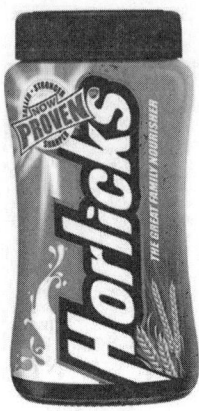

Calories	189	Sodium	1 mg
Fat	4 g	Potassium	0 mg
Saturated	3 g	Carbohydrates	27 g
Sugars	19 g	Protein	10 g
Cholesterol	0 mg	Vitamin A	36%
Calcium	88%	Vitamin C	28%
Iron	19		

ICE CREAM CONES

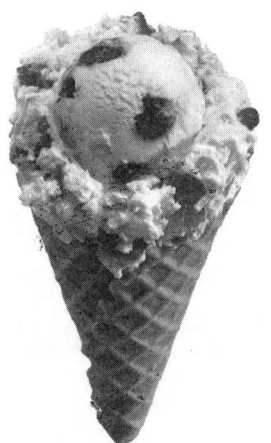

1 cone	
Calories	40
Fat	0.38 g
Saturated fat	0.057 g
Polyunsaturated fat	0.145 g
Monounsaturated fat	0.147 g
Sodium	32 mg
Potassium	14 mg
Carbohydrate	8.41 g
Dietary fiber	0.2 g
Sugars	2.57 g
Protein	0.79 g

CHOCOLATE ICE CREAM CONE

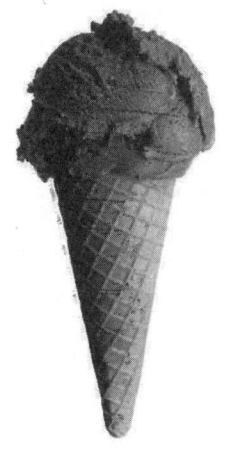

1 cone	
Calories	173
Fat	7.43 g
Saturated fat	4.405 g
Polyunsaturated fat	0.455 g
Monounsaturated fat	2.144 g
Cholesterol	18 mg
Sodium	45 mg
Potassium	168 mg
Carbohydrateohydrate	24.77 g
Dietary fiber	0.8 g
Sugars	19.64 g
Protein	3.18 g

ICE CREAM CHOCOLATE

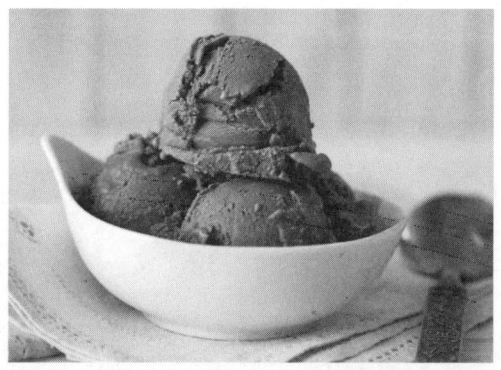

100 gm			
Calories	216	Fat	11 g
Saturated fat	7 g	Polyunsaturated fat	0.4 g
Monounsaturated fat	3.2 g	Cholesterol	34 mg
Sodium	76 mg	Potassium	249 mg
Carbohydrateohydrate	28 g	Dietary fiber	1.2 g
Sugar	25 g	Protein	3.8 g
Caffeine	3 mg		

VANILLA ICE CREAM

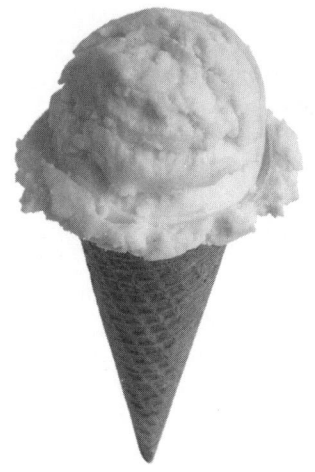

1 cone	
Calories	145
Fat	7.92 g
Saturated fat	4.889 g
Polyunsaturated fat	0.325 g
Monounsaturated fat	2.138 g
Cholesterol	32 mg
Sodium	58 mg
Potassium	143 mg
Carbohydrate	16.99 g
Dietary fiber	0.5 g
Sugars	15.28 g

DAIRY MILK CHOCOLATES

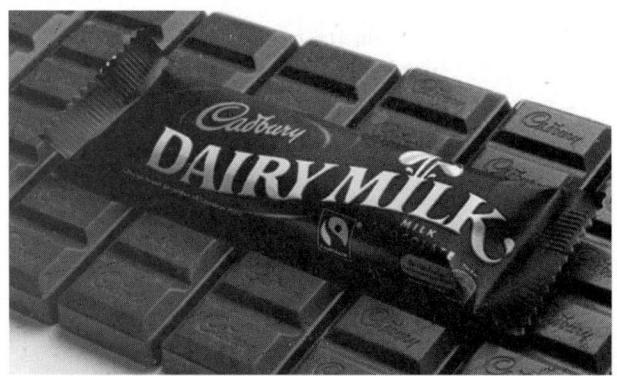

10 blocks (40 g)			
Calories	220	Fat	12.0 g
Saturated fat	8.0 g	Cholesterol	10 mg
Sodium	45 mg	Carbohydrates	24.0 g
Dietary fiber	1.0 g	Sugar	21.0 g
Protein	3.0 g		

CURD

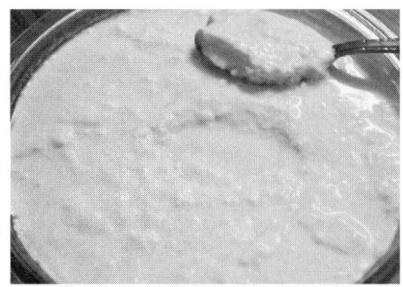

Per 100 ml			
Calories	98	Fat	4.3 g
Saturated fat	1.7 g	Polyunsaturated fat	0.1 g
Monounsaturated fat	0.8 g	Cholesterol	17 mg
Sodium	364 mg	Potassium	104 mg
Carbohydrateohydrate	3.4 g	Dietary fiber	0 g
Sugar	2.7 g	Protein	11 g

- Low in fat.
- Healthy for high cholesterol persons.
- For skin gives glow and softness.
- Cures inflammatory diseases.
- Boost up immune system.
- Rich in high calcium
- Useful in dysentery, vaginal infections and high blood pressure.
- Helps in gaining weight.

YOGURT

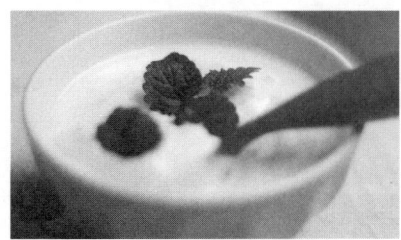

Per 100 gm			
Energy	61 kcal	Carbohydrates	4.7 g
Sugars	4.7 gm	Fat	3.3 g
Saturated	2.1 g	Monounsaturated	0.9 g
Protein	3.5 g	Vitamin A	27 µg
Riboflavin	0.14 mg	Calcium	121 mg

- Rich in protein, calcium, riboflavin, vitamin B_6 and vitamin B_{12}.
- Preventing antibiotic-associated diarrhea.
- Valuable health food for both infants and elderly persons.
- Balanced source of protein, fats, carbohydrates, and minerals.
- Prevents osteoporosis, reduces the risk of high blood pressure and vaginal infections.

BUTTER

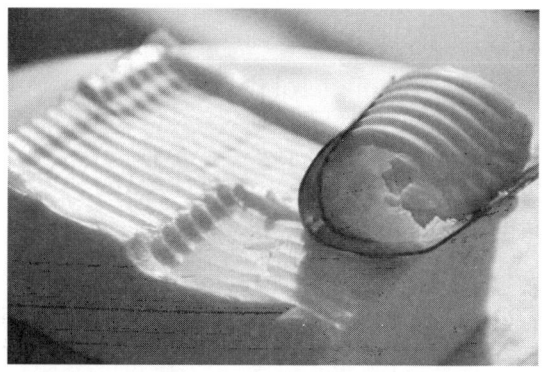

Per 100 gm			
Fat	81 g	Saturated fat	51 g
Polyunsaturated fat	3 g	Monounsaturated fat	21 g
Trans fat	3.3 g	Cholesterol	215 mg
Sodium	11 mg	Potassium	24 mg
Carbohydrateohydrate	0.1 g	Dietary fiber	0 g
Sugar	0.1 g	Protein	0.8 g

- Excellent source of vitamins A, D, E and K.
- Rich in manganese, chromium, iodine, zinc, copper and selenium.
- Rich in healthy fatty acids both short and medium-chain fatty acids which boost up immune system and metabolism.
- Rich in good cholesterol.
- Contains Wulzen factor—which prevents arthritis.
- Have perfect balance of omega-3 and omega-6 fats which helps in brain function, skin health and prostaglandin balance.
- Rich in conjugated linoleic acid which protects against malignancies.
- Contains glycosphingolipids which protects the stomach from gastrointestinal infections.

DARK CHOCOLATE—THEOBROMA CACAO TREE

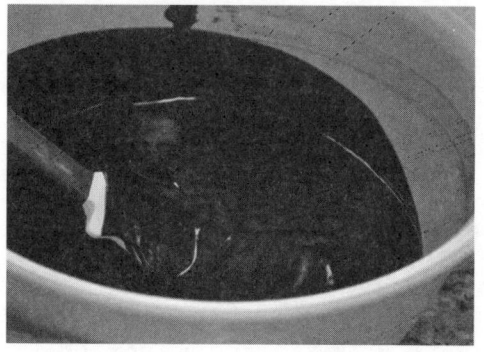

Per 100 gm			
Calories	546	Fat	31 g
Saturated fat	19 g	Polyunsaturated fat	1.1 g
Monounsaturated fat	10 g	Trans fat	0.1 g
Cholesterol	8 mg	Sodium	24 mg

- Lowers blood pressure, improves blood flow and prevents formation of blood clots also prevent arteriosclerosis.
- Increases blood flow to the brain as well as to the heart, so improves cognitive function and reduces risk of stroke.

- Contains theobromine which harden tooth enamel, lowers risk of getting cavities.
- Rich in potassium, copper, magnesium and iron.
- Contains phenylethylamine, it improves mood and makes happier.
- Contains caffeine, a mild stimulant.
- Controls blood sugar.
- Protect against type 2 diabetes.
- Has low glycemic index.
- Rich in antioxidants which protects against malignancy and slows the signs of aging.

WHITE CHOCOLATE

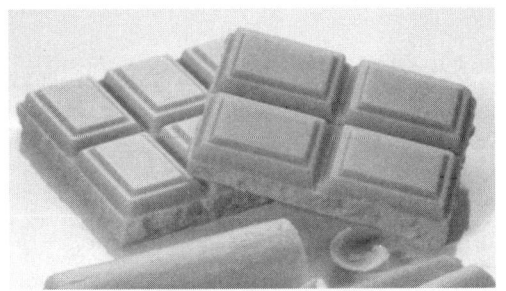

Per 100 gm			
Energy (kJ)	2260	Protein	7.5 g
Lipids	37 g	Carbohydrates	52 g
Lecithin	0.3 g	Theobromine	
Calcium	250 mg	Magnesium	30 mg
Phosphorus	200 mg	Iron	traces
Copper	traces	Vitamin A	220 IU
Vitamin B$_1$	0.1 mg	Vitamin B$_2$	0.4 mg
Vitamin C	3 mg	Vitamin D	15 IU
Vitamin E	traces		

- Source of empty.
- Lots of sugar and saturated fat.
- Rich in riboflavin, calcium and phosphorus.
- Caffeine free.

CHOCOLATE CAKE WITH CHOCOLATE FROSTING

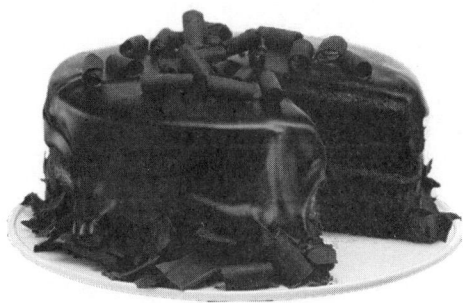

1 piece (1/8 of 18 oz cake)			
Calories	235	Fat	10.5 g
Saturated fat	3.053 g	Polyunsaturated fat	1.181 g
Monounsaturated fat	5.606 g	Cholesterol	27 mg
Sodium	214 mg	Potassium	128 mg
Carbohydrateohydrate	34.94 g	Dietary fiber	1.8 g
Protein	2.62 g		

BOVINE COLOSTRUM

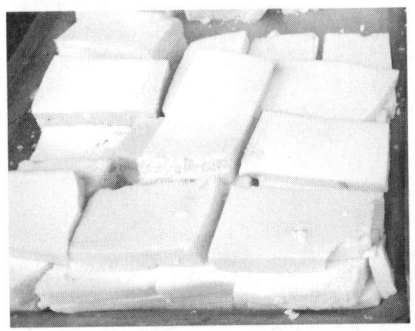

1 cup/8 fl. oz (8 oz)			
Calories	160	Fat	9 g
Saturated fat	6 g	Cholesterol	40 mg
Sodium	120 mg 5%	Carbohydrate	9 g
Dietary fiber	4 g	Sugars	2.4 g
Protein	10 g		

- It is a super food.
- Rich in immunoglobulins.
- Rich in IGF-1, useful of a weight reduction and with dementia
- Rich in amino acids, antioxidants, variety of proteins, vitamins and minerals.
- Contains IGF-1 and IGF-2 insulin-like growth factors which increases growth of muscle fibers and tissues.
- Contains antioxidant-lactoferrin and hemopexin which binds free heme in the body.
- Has great benefits for athletes.

Goat colostrom:
- Yellowish, thick and sticky.
- High in nutrients, antibodies and protein.
- Low in fat.
- "Liquid gold."
- Rich in vitamins A, E and iron.
- Contains antibodies against bacteria and disease.

HONEY

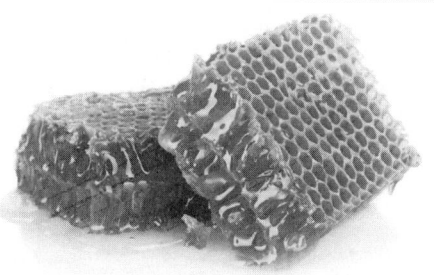

Per 100 gm			
Energy	304 kcal	Carbohydrates	82.4 g
Sugars	82.12 g	Dietary fiber	0.2 g
Fat	0 g	Protein	0.3 g
Calcium	6 mg	Iron	0.42 mg
Magnesium	2 mg	Phosphorus	4 mg
Potassium	52 mg	Sodium	4 mg
Zinc	0.22 mg	Riboflavin	0.038 mg
Niacin	0.121 mg	Pantothenic acid	0.068 mg
Vitamin B_6	0.024 mg	Folic acid	2 µg
Vitamin C	0.5 mg		

- Low in calories and fat.
- Has laxative effect relief from constipation.
- Useful in treatment of persistent coughs, sore throat, diarrhea, dysentery, burns, infected surgical wounds and ulcers.
- Useful for anemia, asthma, baldness, fatigue, headaches, high blood pressure, infertility, insect bites, insomnia, osteoporosis, paralysis, stress and tuberculosis.
- Have anti-bacterial properties.
- Improving appetite.
- Prevents wrinkles on face.

SUGAR-GRANULATED

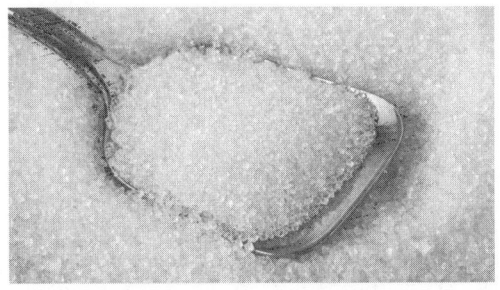

Energy	387 kcal	Carbohydrates	99.98 g
Sugars	99.91 g	Dietary fiber	0 g
Fat	0 g	Protein	0 g
Water	0.03 g	Riboflavin	0.019 mg
Calcium	1 mg	Iron	0.01 mg
Potassium	2 mg		

Types of Sugar

Monosaccharides:
- Glucose, dextrose (fruits and plant).
- Fructose (fruits, root vegetables, cane sugar and honey).
- Galactose (milk sugar).

Disaccharides:
- Sucrose (stems of sugar cane and roots of sugar beet).
- Maltose (germination of barley) lactose (milk).

Side effects:

- Depresses immune system.
- Increases triglyceride, adrenaline and insulin level.
- Also leads to chromium and copper deficiencies.
- Increased risk for cardiovascular disease, Alzheimer's disease, macular degeneration.
- Chances of sugar addiction.
- Hyperactivity in children.
- Promotes obesity, tooth decay and depression, risk of diabetes, heart disease, high blood pressure and cholesterol.

SUGARS, BROWN

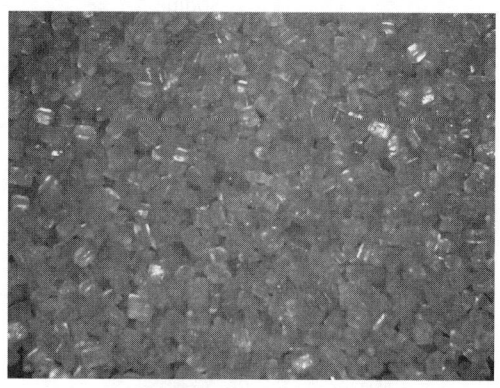

Per 100 gm			
Energy	377 kcal	Carbohydrates	97.33 g
Sugars	96.21 g	Dietary fiber	0 g
Fat	0 g	Protein	0 g
Water	1.77 g	Thiamine	0.008 mg
Riboflavin	0.007 mg	Niacin	0.082 mg
Vitamin B_6	0.026 mg	Folic acid	1 µg
Calcium	85 mg	Iron	1.91 mg
Magnesium	29 mg	Phosphorus	22 mg
Potassium	133 mg	Sodium	39 mg
Zinc	0.18 mg		

JAGGERY

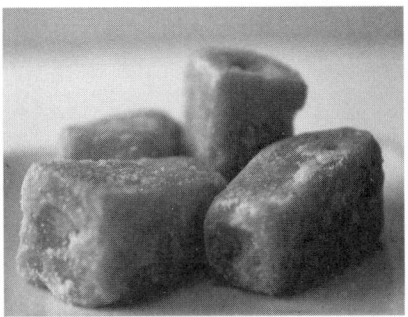

Per 100 gm			
Calories	383	Sodium	27 mg
Fat	0 g	Potassium	453 mg
Saturated	0 g	Carbohydrates	95 g
Sugars	46 g	Protein	0 g
Iron	2.6 gm	Calcium	80 mg

ROCK SUGAR (KHADI SAKHAR)

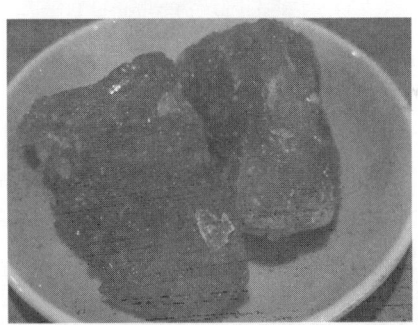

Per tsp	
Calories	25

- Higher in calories.
- American Heart Association recommends women limit consumption of added sugars to 100 calories per day and men limit theirs to 150 calories per day.

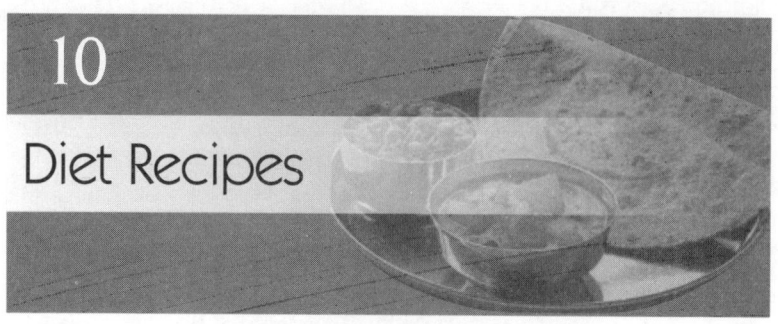

10
Diet Recipes

CHAPATTI

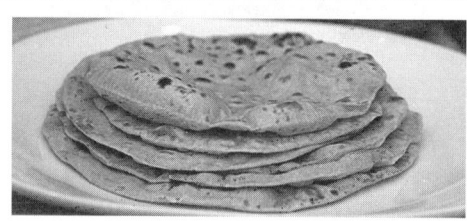

	1 Roti		
Calories	140	Fat	8 g
Carbs	17 g	Protein	3 g

POTATO SABZI (BHAAJI)

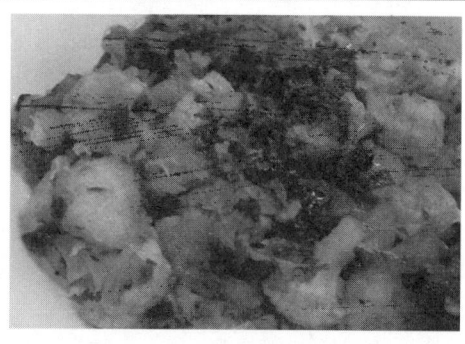

Calories	68	Fat	0.08 g
Carbs	15.7 g	Protein	1.46 g

CABBAGE SABZI

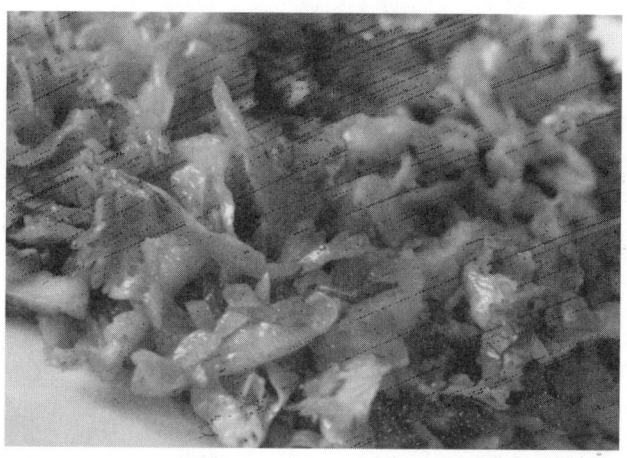

| Calories | 83 | Fat | 4.9 g |
| Carbs | 9.3 g | Protein | 2.6 g |

CAULIFLOWER SABZI

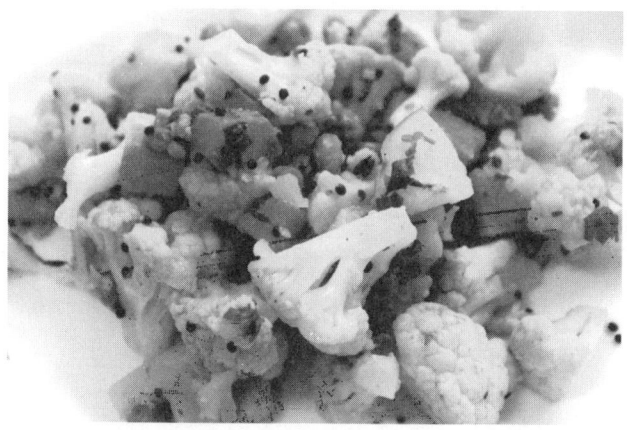

| Calories | 62 | Fat | 4.28 g |
| Carbs | 5.2 g | Protein | 2.3 g |

VEGETABLE CURRY

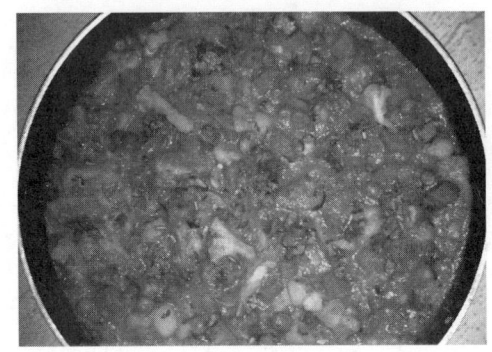

200 gm			
Calories	190	Fat	8.0 g
Sodium	1610 mg	Carbohydrates	26.0 g
Protein	4.0 g	Kidney beans (rajma) [usal]	
Calories	225	Fat	0.88 g
Carbs	40.36 g	Protein	15.35 g
Black eye peas(chavali) [usal]		Energy	225 cal
Fat	0.88 g	Carbs	40.36 g
Protein	15.35 g		

KIDNEY BEANS(RAJMA) [USAL]

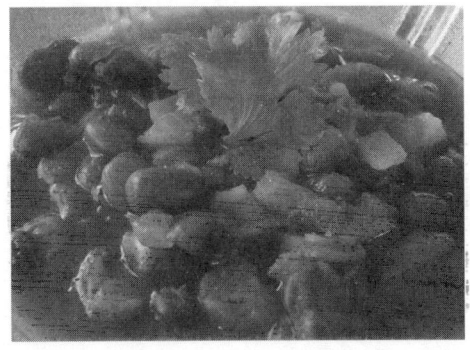

Calories	225	Fat	0.88 g
Carbs	40.36 g	Protein	15.35 g

BLACK EYE PEAS(CHAVALI) [USAL]

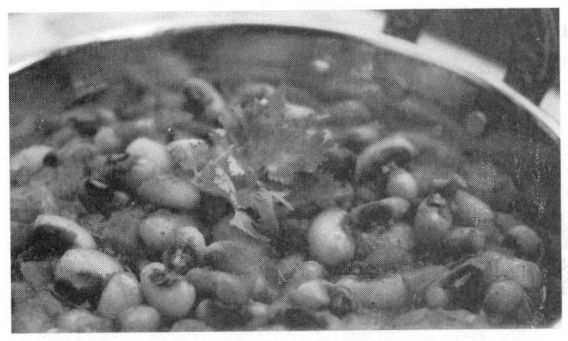

| Energy | 225 cal | Fat | 0.88 g |
| Carbs | 40.36 g | Protein | 15.35 g |

SOYA BEAN

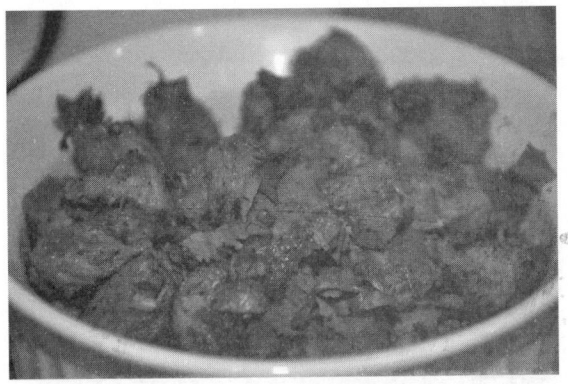

Calories	149	Sodium	204 mg
Fat	8 g	Potassium	0 mg
Saturated	1 g	Carbs	9 g
Polyunsaturated	4 g	Dietary fiber	5 g
Monounsaturated	2 g	Sugars	3 g
Protein	14 g		

MANGO PICKLE

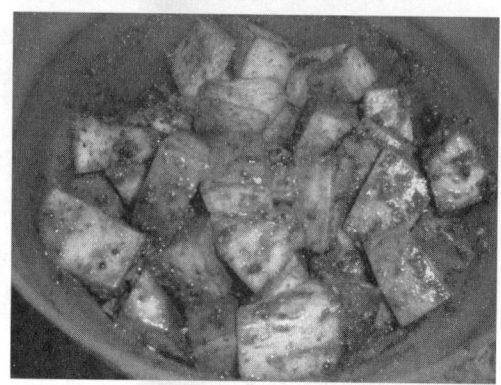

	1 tbsp (15 gm)		
Calories	25	Fat	1.5 g
Cholesterol	0 mg	Sodium	960 mg
Carbohydrates	2.0 g	Dietary fiber	1.0 g
Protein	0.0 g		

PURAN POLI

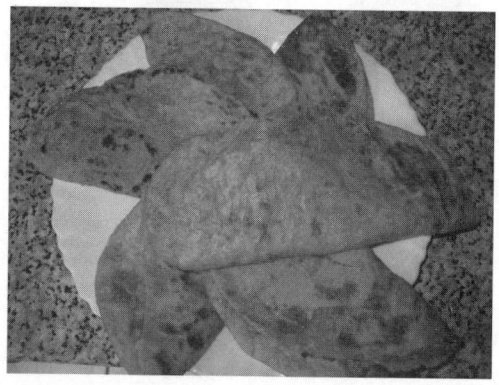

Channa dal or split yellow gram	300 gm
Jaggery or sugar	300 gm
Cardamom powder, nutmeg powder	1 tsp
Plain flour	150 gm

11

Milk of Mammals

HUMAN BREAST MILK

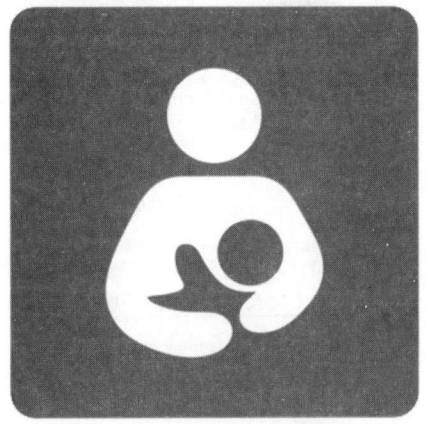

		100 ml	
Fat	4.2 gm	Protein	1.1 gm
Casein	0.4	α-lactalbumin	0.3
Lactoferrin	0.2	IgA	0.1
(apo-lactoferrin)		IgG	0.001
Lysozyme	0.05	Serum albumin	0.05
Carbohydrate	(g/100 ml)	Lactose	7
Oligosaccharides	0.5	Calcium	0.03
Phosphorus	0.014	Sodium	0.015
Potassium	0.055	Chlorine	0.043

- Contains strong antibodies and antitoxins.
- Home remedy for minor ailments, such as conjunctivitis, insect bites and stings, contact dermatitis, and infected wounds, burns, and abrasions.
- Breast milk boosts up immunity.

Benefits Against Diseases

- Lowered risk of Sudden Infant Death Syndrome (SIDS).
- Increased intelligence.
- Decreased middle ear infections, cold and flu resistance.
- A decrease in the risk of childhood leukemia.
- Lower risk of childhood onset diabetes.
- Decreased risk of asthma and eczema.
- Decreased risk of obesity, autism, and decreased risk of developing psychological disorders.

Milk Volume

- From birth to 24 hours, colostrum averages about 37 ml.
- From 24 to 96 hours, there is a slow rise in volume.
- Day 5: Approximately 500 ml/day.
- 3 to 5 months: 750 ml/day.
- 6 months: 800 ml/day.

COW MILK

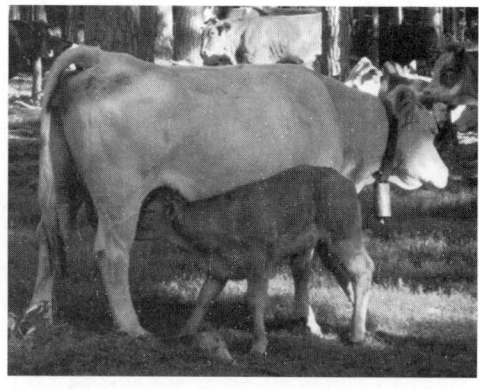

1 cup			
Carbohydrate	11.71 g	Protein	8.13 g
Fat	6.68 g	Saturated fat	2.92 g
Citric acid	512.40 mg	Calories	212.20
Sugar total	11.71 g	Vitamin A IU	500.20 IU
Thiamin-B$_1$	0.10 mg	Riboflavin-B$_2$	0.40 mg
Niacin-B$_3$	0.21 mg	Vitamin B$_6$	0.10 mg
Vitamin B$_{12}$	0.89 mcg	Biotin	4.88 mcg
Vitamin C	2.32 mg	Vitamin D IU	97.60 IU
Vitamin D	2.44 mcg	Folic acid	12.44 mcg
Vitamin K	9.76 mcg	Pantothenic acid	0.78 mg
Calcium	296.70 mg	Chloride	244.00 mg
Copper	0.02 mg	Iodine	58.56 mcg
Iron	0.12 mg	Magnesium	33.35 mg
Phosphorous	232.04 mg	Potassium	376.74 mg
Sodium	121.76 mg	Zinc	0.95 mg
Cholesterol	14 mg		

- Highly nutritious food.
- Rich in calcium, potassium, vitamins and protein.
- Beneficial in the growth and development of bones.
- Beneficial against diseases like gout, kidney stones, breast malignancy, rheumatoid arthritis, migraine headaches.

SKIM MILK

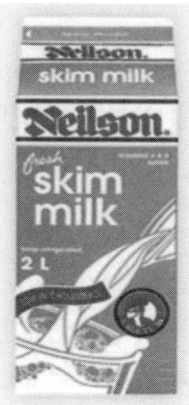

Per cup 8 fl oz			
Calories	80	Fat	0.0 g
Protein	16 g	Carbohydrate	12 g
Cholesterol	10 mg	Sodium	120 mg
Vitamin A	20.000 ~ IU	Vitamin D	2.5 mcg
Vitamin C	8 mcg	Riboflavin	0.3 mg
Vitamin B$_{12}$	0.9 mcg	Calcium	60 mg
Phosphorus	248 mg		

- Less fat.
- Rich in calcium.
- Good amount of energy.
- Ideal for dieting to lose weight.

BUFFALO MILK

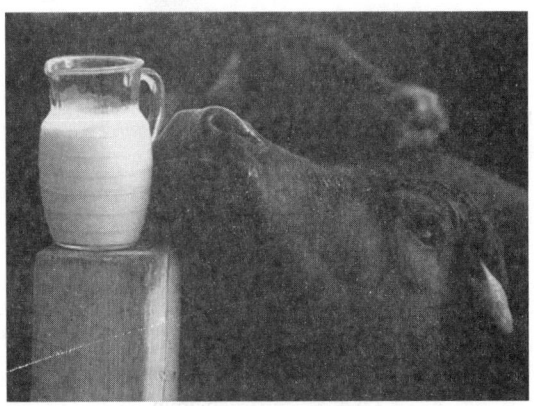

Per 100 gm			
Energy	117.0 cal	Protein	4.3 gm
Minerals	0.8 gm	Carbohydrates	5.0 gm
Calcium	210.00 mg	Phosphorous	130.0 mg
Iron	0.2 mg	Carotene	160.0 µg
Thiamine	0.04 mg	Vitamin B$_{12}$	0.1 µg
Folic acid	3.3 µg	Vitamin C	1.0 mg
Sodium	19.0 mg	Potassium	90.0 mg
Fat	7.97 gm	Cholesterol	0.014 gm

- Perfect food.
- High in protein, calcium, phosphorus, vitamin A, thiamine, riboflavin and nicotinic acid.
- Poor in vitamins C and E.
- Contains vitamin B_{12}.
- Low in cholesterol.

SHEEP MILK

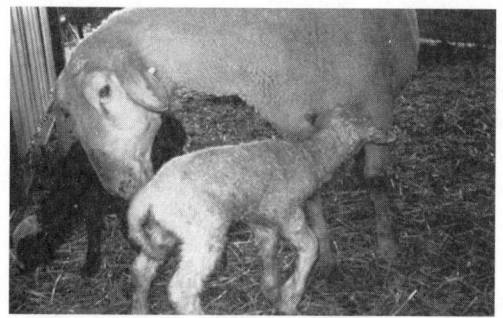

Per 100 gm			
Energy	108 kcal	Protein	5.98 gm
Lipids [fat]	7.01 gm	Carbohydrate	5.36 gm
Calcium	193 mg	Iron	0.1 mg
Magnesium	18 mg	Phosphorus	158 mg
Potassium	137 mg	Sodium	44 mg
Zinc	0.54 mg	Copper	0.046 mg
Manganese	0.018 mg	Selenium	1.7 mg
Vitamin C	4.2 mg	Thiamin	0.065 mg
Riboflavin	0.355 mg	Niacin	0.417 mg
Pantothenic acid	0.407 mg	Vitamin B_6	0.06 mg
Folic acid	7 mcg	Vitamin B_{12}	0.71 mcg
Vitamin A	147 IU	Cholesterol	27 mg

- Highly nutritious.
- Rich in vitamins A, B, E, calcium, phosphorus, potassium and magnesium.
- Rich in short and medium-chain fatty acids.
- Contains more conjugated linoleic acid.

DONKEY MILK (OR ASS MILK)

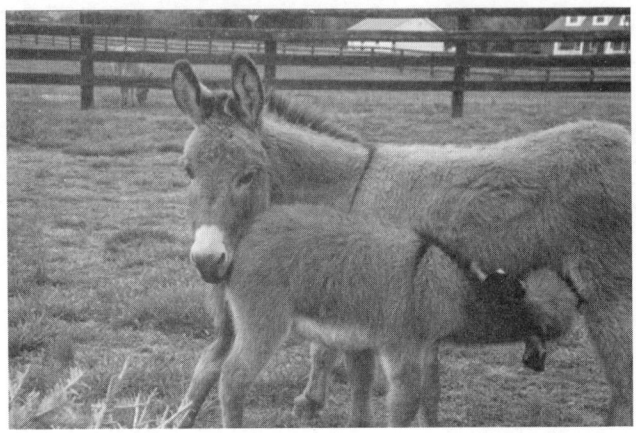

	Per 100 gm		
pH	7.0–7.2	Protein	1.5–1.8 gm
Fat	0.3–1.8 gm	Lactose	5.8–7.4 gm
Whey protein	0.49–0.80 gm		

- Similar to human breast milk.
- Poor in protein and fat.
- Rich in lactose.
- Effective in preventing wrinkles on face and makes skin more delicate.
- Used in the manufacture of soaps and moisturizers.
- Relieves constipation
- Folk belief that this milk boost up infants' immunity and voice development.
- Cures liver troubles, infectious diseases, fevers, edema, nose bleeds, poisonings and wounds.
- Useful in treatment of poisonings, fever, fatigue, eye strains, asthma and gynecological diseases.

MOOSE MILK, ALSO KNOWN AS ELK MILK

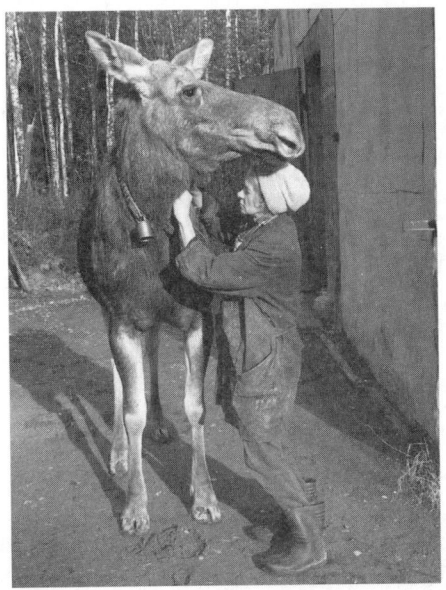

- High in butterfat.
- Higher concentrations of solids.
- Rich in aluminium, iron, selenium and zinc.

CAMEL'S MILK

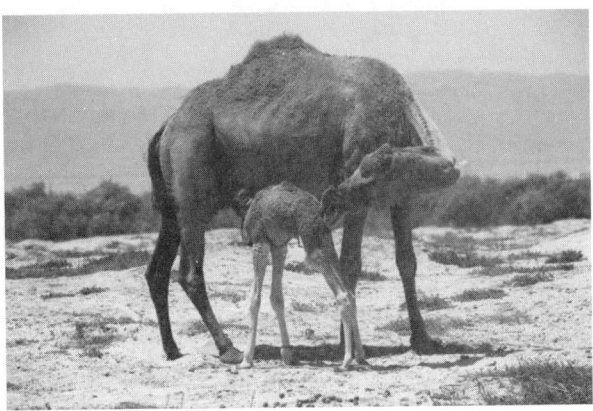

- High vitamin and mineral content and immunoglobin content.
- Low in lactose, vitamins A and B_2.
- Rich in potassium, magnesium, iron, copper, manganese, and sodium.
- Low in cholesterol.
- Contains antibodies against malignancy, HIV, Alzheimer's disease and hepatitis B. High concentration of insulin to control diabetes blood sugar levels.
- Helps in reducing coronary heart disease.
- Higher in vitamin C, unsaturated fatty acids and B vitamins.
- Slightly saltier.

WHALE MILK

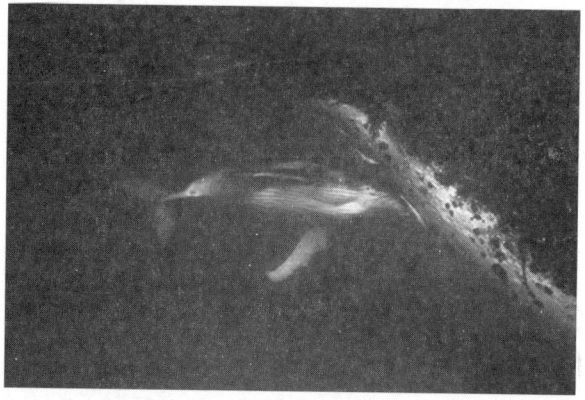

- Largest animal.
- Nurse their young with milk from mammary glands.
- Whale cows nurse by actively squirting milk into the mouths of their young.
- 35–50% high fat percentage.
- Whales milk travel through the water without breaking up.
- Toothpaste like consistency.

CAT MILK

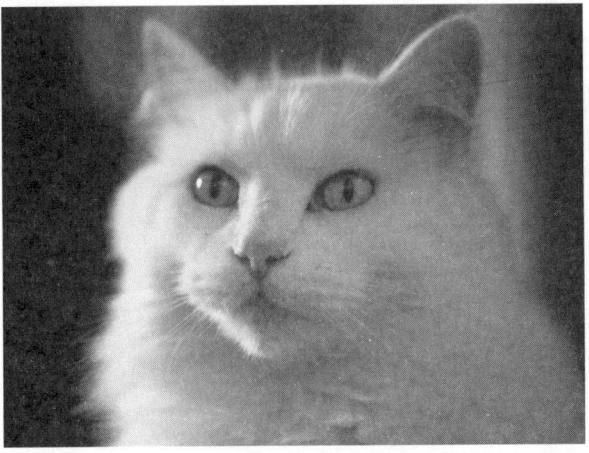

| Fat | 10.8% | Protein | 10.6% | Sugar | 3.7% |

- Indescribably creamy
- High butterfat content
- Slight yellow color

12

Miscellaneous Nutrition

LEMON GRASS—CYMBOPOGON

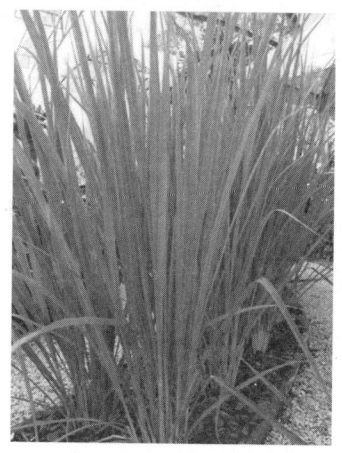

Per 100 gm			
Energy	99 kcal	Carbohydrates	25.31 g
Protein	1.82 g	Fat	0.49 g
Cholesterol	0 mg	Sodium	6 mg
Potassium	723 mg	Calcium	65 mg
Copper	0.266 mg	Iron	8.17 mg
Magnesium	60 mg	Manganese	5.244 mg
Selenium	0.7 µg	Zinc	2.23 mg
Folic acid	75 µg	Niacin	1.101 mg
Pyridoxine	0.080 mg	Riboflavin	0.135 mg
Thiamin	0.065 mg	Vitamin A	6 mg
Vitamin C	2.6 mg		

- Has antioxidant and disease preventing properties.
- Contains citral or lemonal which gives lemon odor and act as anti-microbial and anti-fungal.
- Contains essential oils—myrcene, citronellol, methyl heptenone, dipentene, geraniol, limonene, geranyl acetate and nerol. These act as irritant, rubefacient, insecticidal, anti-fungal and antiseptic.
- Commonly used in herbal teas.
- Relieves colitis, indigestion, gastro-enteritis, sore throats, laryngitis, bronchitis.
- Oil is used in massage therapy as a muscle and skin-toner.
- Rich in folic acid which prevents neural tube defects in the baby.
- Rich in pantothenic acid, pyridoxine and thiamin.
- Contains vitamins C and A.
- Rich in potassium, zinc, calcium, iron, manganese, copper, and magnesium.

SHATAVARI (ASPARAGUS RACEMOSUS)

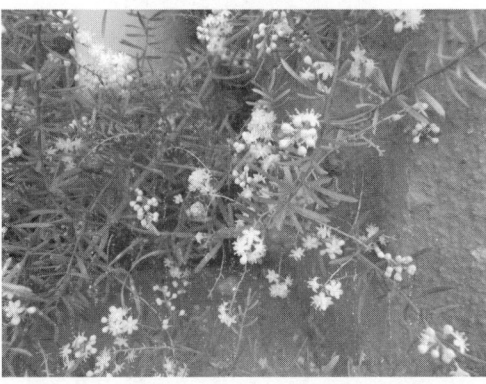

- Word meaning—she who possesses a hundred husbands.
- Also known as "woman's best friend" or "queen of herbs."
- Useful in treating infertility, both male and female, for regulating ovulation, and relieves symptoms of menstruation.

- Useful against malignancy, cough, diarrhea, dehydration, dysentry, chronic fever, bronchitis, hyperacidity, herpes, impotence, infertility, AIDS, lung abscess, muscle spasms, menopause, rheumatism, stiffness of joints, and stomach ulcers.
- Also used for increasing lactation in nursing mothers.
- Is diuretic, antispasmodic, aphrodisiac and a nutritive tonic.

BASIL (TULSA)

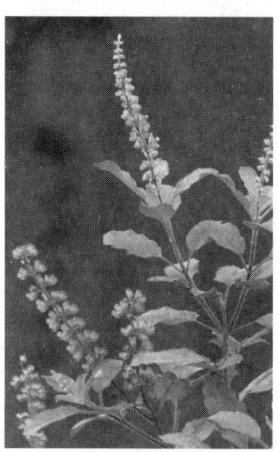

Per 100 gm			
Energy	22 kcal	Carbohydrates	2.65 g
Dietary fiber	1.6 g	Fat	0.64 g
Protein	3.15 g	Vitamin A	264 µg
Beta-carotene	3142 µg	Thiamine	0.034 mg
Riboflavin	0.076 mg	Niacin	0.902 mg
Pantothenic acid	0.209 mg	Vitamin B_6	0.155 mg
Folic acid	68 µg	Choline	11.4 mg
Vitamin C	18.0 mg	Vitamin E	0.80 mg
Vitamin K	414.8 µg	Calcium	177 mg
Iron	3.17 mg	Magnesium	64 mg
Manganese	1.148 mg	Phosphorus	56 mg
Potassium	295 mg	Sodium	4 mg
Zinc	0.81 mg		

- Contains polyphenolic flavonoids—orientin and vicenin which has antioxidant protection against radiation.
- Contains essential oils—eugenol, citronellol, linalool, citral, limonene and terpineol. These have anti-inflammatory and anti-bacterial properties.
- Low in calories.
- Cholesterol free.
- Rich in beta-carotene, vitamin A, cryptoxanthin, lutein and zeaxanthin.
- Contains zeaxanthin and vitamin A which prevents from lung and oral cavity malignancies.
- Rich in vitamin K, potassium, manganese, copper, magnesium and iron.
- It reduces blood pressure.
- Boosts up the immune system.
- Inhibits growth HIV and carcinogenic cells.
- Prevents cataract, macular degeneration, and glaucoma and vision defects.
- Also useful in reducing labor pain, destroying rabies germs, treating gastroenteritis, cholera, whooping cough and destroying worms.
- Destroys more than 99 per cent of the germs and bacteria in the mouth, so excellent mouth freshener and oral disinfectant.
- Relieves pain of kidney stones.
- Useful in migraine, sinus, cough and cold, high blood pressure, etc.
- Prevents signs of ageing.

FRAGRANT CINNAMON "QUILL."

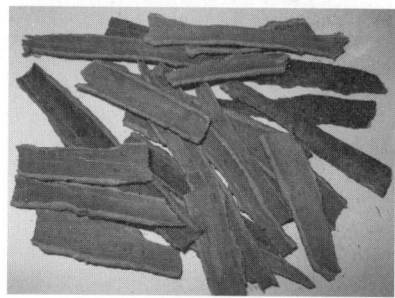

Energy	247 kcal	Carbohydrates	50.59 g
Protein	3.99 g	Fat	1.24 g
Cholesterol	0 mg	Dietary fiber	53.1 g
Sodium	10 mg	Potassium	431 mg
Calcium	1002 mg	Copper	0.339 mg
Iron	8.32 mg	Magnesium	60 mg
Manganese	17.466 mg	Phosphorus	64 mg
Zinc	1.83 mg	Folic acid	6 µg
Niacin	1.332 mg	Pantothenic acid	0.358 mg
Pyridoxine	0.158 mg	Riboflavin	0.041 mg
Thiamin	0.022 mg	Vitamin A	295 IU
Vitamin C	3.8 mg	Vitamin E	10.44 mg
Vitamin K	31.2 µg		

- Highly prized spices.

- Has antioxidant, anti-diabetic, antiseptic, local anesthetic, anti-inflammatory, rubefacient (warming and soothing), carminative and anti-flatulent properties.

- Contains eugenol-acid which gives pleasant, sweet aromatic fragrances. Eugenol has got local anesthetic and antiseptic properties, hence useful in dental and gum treatment procedures.

- Essential oils in cinnamon include ethyl cinnamate, linalool, cinnamaldehyde, beta-caryophyllene, and methyl chavicol.

- Anti-clotting action, prevents platelet clogging inside the blood vessels, and thereby helps prevent stroke, peripheral arterial and coronary artery diseases.

- Increases the motility of the intestinal tract as well as help aid in the digestion power by increasing gastro-intestinal enzyme secretions.

- Excellent source of potassium, calcium, manganese, iron, zinc, and magnesium.

- Rich in vitamin A, niacin, pantothenic acid, and pyridoxine.

CHILI PEPPERS

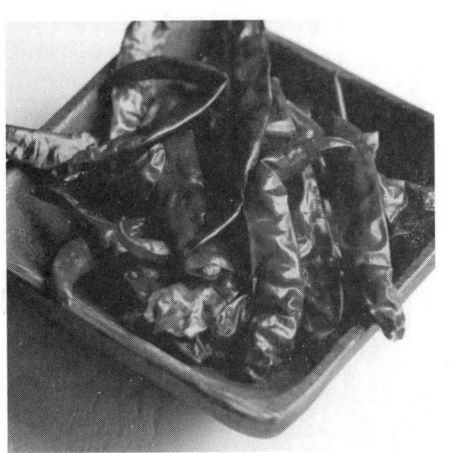

		Per 100 gm	
Energy	40 kcal	Carbohydrates	8.81 g
Protein	1.87 g	Fat	0.44 g
Cholesterol	0 mg	Dietary fiber	1.5 g
Sodium	9 mg	Potassium	322 mg
Calcium	14 mg	Copper	0.129 mg
Iron	1.03 mg	Magnesium	23 mg
Manganese	0.187 mg	Phosphorus	43 mg
Selenium	0.5 µg	Zinc	0.26 mg
Folic acid	23 µg	Niacin	1.244 mg
Pantothenic acid	0.201 mg	Pyridoxine	0.506 mg
Riboflavin	0.086 mg	Thiamin	0.72 mg
Vitamin A	952 IU	Vitamin C	143.7 mg
Vitamin E	0.69 mg	Vitamin K	14 µg

- Contains alkaloid compound—capsaicin which has anti-bacterial, anti-carcinogenic, analgesic and anti-diabetic properties.
- Reduces LDL cholesterol levels in obese individuals.
- Rich in potassium, manganese, iron, and magnesium.
- Rich in niacin, pyridoxine riboflavin and thiamin.
- Cholesterol free.

- Rich source of vitamin C.
- Contains vitamin A, and flavonoids like β-carotene, α-carotene, lutein, zeaxanthin, and cryptoxanthin.

CARAWAY SEED

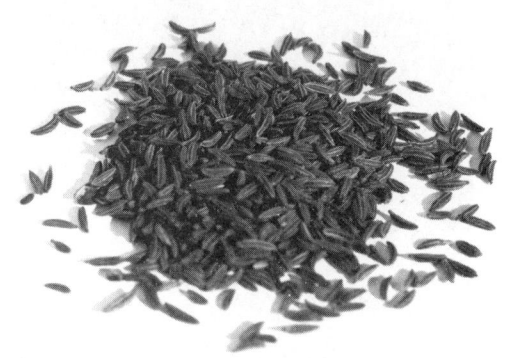

Per 100 gm			
Energy	333 kcal	Carbohydrates	49.90 g
Protein	19.77 g	Fat	14.59 g
Cholesterol	0 mg	Dietary fiber	38 g
Sodium	17 mg	Potassium	1351 mg
Calcium	689 mg	Copper	0.910 mg
Iron	16.23 mg	Magnesium	258 mg
Manganese	1.300 mg	Phosphorus	568 mg
Zinc	5.5 mg	Folic acid	10 µg
Niacin	3.606 mg	Pyridoxine	0.360 mg
Riboflavin	0.379 mg	Thiamin	0.383 mg
Vitamin A	363 IU	Vitamin C	21 mg
Vitamin E	2.5 mg		

- Rich source of dietary fiber.
- Lowers serum LDL cholesterol levels.
- Rich in iron, copper, calcium, potassium, manganese, selenium, zinc and magnesium.
- Rich in vitamin A, vitamin E, vitamin C, thiamin, pyridoxine, riboflavin, and niacin.

- Contains essential oils—carvone, limonene, carveol, pinen, cumuninic aldehyde, furfurol and thujone. These are anti-oxidant, digestive, carminative and anti-flatulent properties.
- Contains flavonoid antioxidnats like lutein, carotene, crypto-xanthin and zeaxanthin. These protects from malignancies, infection, aging and degenerative neurological diseases.

CAPERS

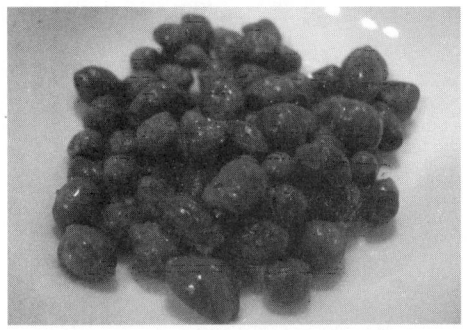

Per 100 gm			
Energy	23 kcal	Carbohydrates	4.89 g
Protein	2.36 g	Fat	0.86 g
Cholesterol	0 mg	Dietary fiber	3.2 g
Sodium	2954 mg	Potassium	40 mg
Calcium	40 mg	Copper	0.374 mg
Iron	1.67 mg	Magnesium	33 mg
Manganese	0.078 mg	Phosphorus	10 mg
Selenium	1.2 mcg	Zinc	0.32 mg
Folic acid	23 mcg	Niacin	0.652 mg
Pantothenic acid	0.027 mg	Pyridoxine	0.023 mg
Riboflavin	0.139 mg	Thiamin	0.018 mg
Vitamin A	138 IU	Vitamin C	4.3 mg
Vitamin E	0.88 mg	Vitamin K	24.6 mcg

- Very low in calories.
- High in flavonoid-rutin and quercetin which are anti-bacterial, anti-carcinogenic, analgesic and anti-inflammatory action.

- Useful in treatment of hemorrhoids, varicose veins and hemophilia.
- Relieves rheumatic pain.
- Acts as appetite stimulant.
- Reduces LDL cholesterol levels in obese individuals.
- Rich in vitamin A, vitamin K, niacin, and riboflavin.
- Rich in calcium, iron, and copper.

BLACK PEPPER

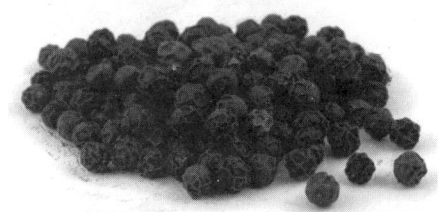

Energy	255 kcal	Carbohydrates	64.81 g
Protein	10.95 g	Fat	3.26 g
Cholesterol	0 mg	Dietary fiber	26.5 g
Choline	11.3 mg	Sodium	44 mg
Potassium	1259 mg	Calcium	437 mg
Copper	1.127 mg	Iron	28.86 mg
Magnesium	194 mg	Manganese	5.625 mg
Phosphorus	173 mg	Zinc	1.42 mg
Folic acid	10 mcg	Niacin	1.142 mg
Pyridoxine	0.340 mg	Riboflavin	0.240 mg
Thiamin	0.109 mg	Vitamin A	299 IU
Vitamin C	21 mg	Vitamin E	4.56 mg
Vitamin K	163.7 mcg		

King of Spice

- Has anti-inflammatory, carminative, anti-flatulent properties.
- Contains essential oils—piperine, which gives strong spicy pungent character.
- Rich in potassium, calcium, zinc, manganese, iron and magnesium.

- Excellent source of pyridoxine, riboflavin, thiamin and niacin.
- Rich in vitamins C and A, which protects from malignancies and diseases.
- Contains monoterpenes hydrocarbons like sabinene, pinene, terpenene, limonene, mercene which gives aromatic property.
- Increases the gut motility as well as the digestion power.

BAY LEAF

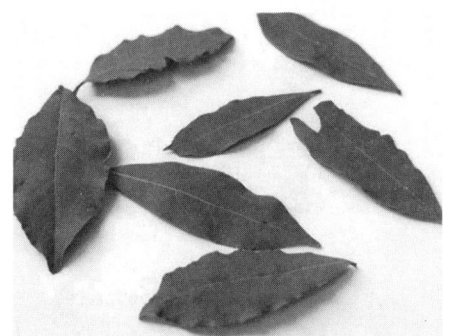

Energy	313 kcal	Carbohydrates	74.97 g
Protein	7.61 g	Fat	8.36 g
Cholesterol	0 mg	Dietary fiber	26.3 g
Sodium	23 mg	Potassium	529 mg
Calcium	834 mg	Copper	0.416 mg
Iron	43 mg	Magnesium	120 mg
Manganese	8.167 mg	Phosphorus	113 mg
Selenium	2.8 mcg	Zinc	3.70 mg
Folic acid	180 mcg	Niacin	2.005 mg
Pyridoxine	1.740 mg	Riboflavin	0.421 mg
Vitamin A	6185 IU	Vitamin C	46.5 mg

- Known as tree of the Sun God.
- Contains α-pinene, β-pinene, myrcene, limonene, linalool, methyl chavicol, neral, α-terpineol, geranyl acetate, eugenol, and chavicol. These are antiseptic, antioxidant, digestive, and anti-malignancy in action.
- Rich in vitamin A which protects from lung and oral cavity malignancies.

- Rich in niacin, pyridoxine, pantothenic acid and riboflavin.
- Good source of copper, potassium, calcium, manganese, iron, selenium, zinc and magnesium.
- It has astringent, diuretic, and appetite stimulant properties.
- Relieves flatulence and colic pain.
- It has insect repellent action.
- Useful in treatment of arthritis, muscle pain, bronchitis and flu symptoms.
- Rich source of vitamin C which is immune booster.
- Rich in folic acid which prevents neural tube defects in the baby.

ALLSPICE

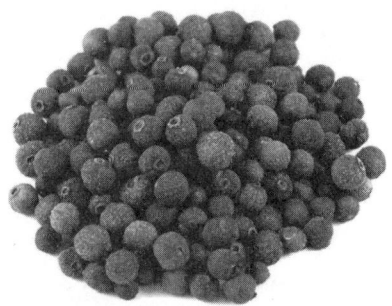

Energy	236 cal	Carbohydrates	72.12 g
Protein	6.09 g	Fat	8.69 g
Cholesterol	0 mg	Dietary fiber	21.6 g
Sodium	77 mg	Potassium	1044 mg
Calcium	661 mg	Copper	0.553 mg
Iron	7.06 mg	Magnesium	135 mg
Manganese	2.943 mg	Phosphorus	113 mg
Zinc	1.01 mg	Folic acid	36 µg
Niacin	2.860 mg	Pantothenic acid	0.210 mg
Pyridoxine	0.210 mg	Riboflavin	0.063 mg
Thiamin	0.101 mg	Vitamin A	540 IU
Vitamin C	39.2 mg		

Jamaican Pepper or Allspice

- Rich in potassium, manganese, iron, copper, selenium, and magnesium.
- Rich in vitamin A, vitamin B_6, riboflavin, niacin and vitamin C.
- Rich in essential oils—eugenol which is pleasant, sweet aromatic fragrances.
- Contains allspice which increases gut motility.
- Has local anesthetic and antiseptic action, so used in gum and dental procedures.
- Useful in flatulence and indigestion in traditional medicine.
- Home remedy for arthritis and sore muscles.

PANCHGAVYA

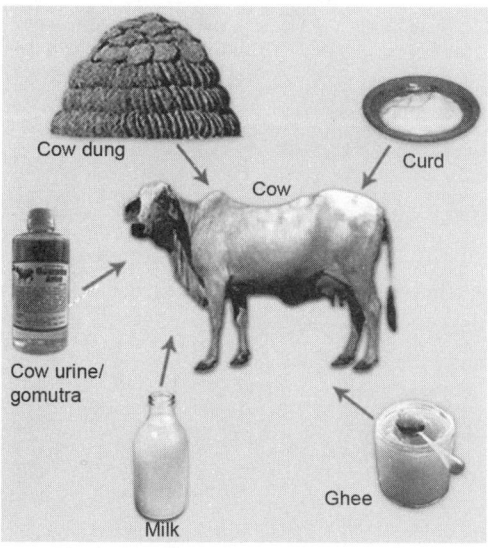

- Five gavya come from Indian COW.
- Cow's urine, dung, milk, curd and ghee.
- Possess medicinal properties
- Distilled cow's urine is potent anti-malignancy and anti-HIV agent.

Uses

- In malignancy.
- High and low blood pressure.
- Heart, kidney, liver diseases.
- Prevents arthritis.
- Useful in dietary and gastrointestinal disorders.
- Useful in asthama, leucoderma hyperlipidemia, diabetes, skin diseases, eye diseases, vitiligo, jaundice, anaemia, tuberculosis, joints pain.

PANCHAMRITA

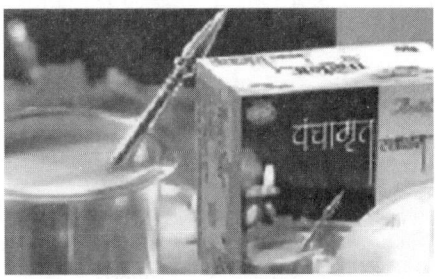

Mixture of Five—Honey, Sugar, Milk, Yogurt, and Ghee

- Milk is for the blessing of purity and piousness.
- Yogurt is for prosperity and progeny.
- Honey is for sweet speech.
- Ghee is for victory.
- Sugar is for happiness.
- Water is for purity.

Cow Urine

- Contains urea-strong antibacterial agent.
- Has strong antibacterial properties which controls malignancy.
- Minerals present are like food—easily absorbed.
- Contains urokinase which dissolves blood clots, helps heart diseases and improves blood circulation.
- Contains epithelium growth factor which helps in regeneration of damaged tissues.

- Promotes production of red blood cells.
- Regulates menstrual cycle and sperm production.
- Contains kallikrin which expands peripheral veins and reduces blood pressure.
- Prevention of muscular tumor.
- Contains anti-neoplaston, h-11 beta-iodole-acetic acid and directine, 3-methyl gloxal. These factors prevents the multiplication of carcinogenic.
- Rich in copper which prevents excessive deposition of fat.
- Rich in iron, potassium, manganese, vitamins A, B, C, D, E.
- Increases vigour and potency.

Galactagogue

A substance that promotes lactation in humans

Domperidone	Torbangun (*Coleus amboinicus lour*)
Metoclopramide	Fennel (*Foeniculum vulgare*)
Risperidone	Milk thistle (*Silybum marianum*)
Chlorpromazine	Chasteberry (*Vitex agnus-castus*)
Sulpiride	Goat's rue (*Galega officinalis*)
Oxytocin	Blessed thistle
Growth hormone	Alfalfa
Thyrotrophin releasing hormone	Anise
Medroxyprogesterone	Nettle
Shatavari (*Asparagus racemosus*)	Oatmeal
Fenugreek (*Trigonella foenum-graecum*)	Vervain
Domperidone	Red raspberry leaf
Metoclopramide	Torbangun (*Coleus amboinicus lour*)
Risperidone	Fennel (*Foeniculum vulgare*)
Chlorpromazine	Milk thistle (*Silybum marianum*)

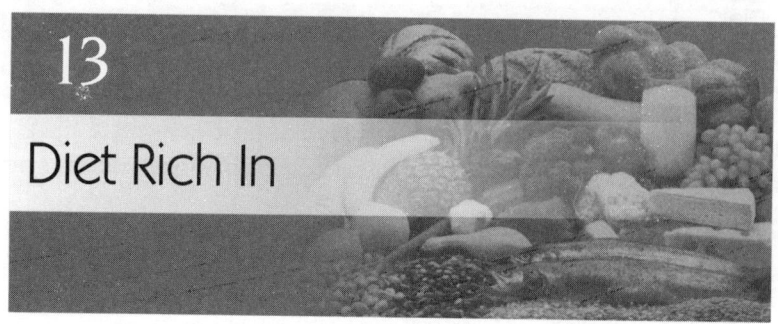

13

Diet Rich In

CALCIUM RICH FRUITS

	Per 100 mg
Dried figs	Rhubarb (cooked)
Dates (medjool)	Kumquats
Prickly pears	Dried apricots
Oranges and tangerines	Prunes (dried plums)
Mulberries	Kiwi (Chinese gooseberries)
Dried figs	

SUGAR RICH FRUITS

	Per 100 gm
Apples	Dates
Amarinds, raw	Apples, dried
Apricots	Papaya
Figs, dried	Bananas
Pineapple juice	

FIBRE RICH FRUITS

	Per 100 gm
Apples	Lemon peel
Orange peel	Bananas
Figs, dried	Dates

PROTEIN RICH FRUITS

Apricots	Bananas
Prunes	Apricots
Figs	Tamarinds
Guavas	Sugar

IRON RICH FRUITS

Apricots, dehydrated	Peaches
Tamarinds	Figs
Apples	

FRUITS RICH IN WATER

	Per 100 gm
	Grapefruit
Apricot	
Watermelon	

FRUITS RICH IN ZINC

Apricots	Peaches
Avocados	Blueberries
Bananas	Apricots
Peaches	Avocados
Blueberries	Bananas

FRUITS HIGH IN CALORIES

	Per 100 gm
	Bananas
Apples	Apricots
Prunes	Apples
Figs, dried	
Plums, dried	

FRUITS RICH IN FAT

Avocados 15.41 g	Olives 15.32 g
Bananas 1.81 g	Pomegranates 1.17 g
Guavas 0.95 g	Figs, dried 0.93 g

COPPER RICH DIET

Per 100 g			
Veal liver	15 mg	Oysters	1–8 mg
Dried sesame seeds	4.1 mg	Cashew nuts	2.2 mg
Sunflower seeds	1.8 mg	Tomato	1.4 mg
Pumpkin and squash seeds	1.4 mg	Dried basil	1.4 mg
Dry roasted soybeans	1.1 mg		

- Copper is an essential mineral required by the body for bone and connective tissue production.
- Deficiency—osteoporosis, joint pain, lowered immunity.
- Over-consumption—cramps, diarrhea, vomiting, depression, schizophrenia, hypertension, senility, and insomnia, poisonous.

CHOLESTEROL LOWERING FOODS

Foods which lowers the "bad" LDL cholesterol, while leaving the good HDL cholesterol:

- Diet rich in niacin
- Exercise
- Become vegan—eating only plant foods reduce stress

Olive oil, canola oil, peanut oil, and avocados oat bran, flax seeds, clove, raw garlic, almonds, red color tomatoes, watermelon, dark non-milk chocolate, green tea.

IRON RICH DIET

Per 100 gm			
Sun-dried tomatoes	9 mg	Dried apricots	6 mg
Fresh parsley	6 mg	Spinach (cooked)	3.5 mg
Dried coconut	3.3 mg	Olives	3.3 mg
Raisins	3 mg	Palm hearts	3 mg
Lentil sprouts	3 mg	Swiss chard	2.3 mg
Broccoli raab	2.1 mg	Figs (dried)	2 mg
Apples (dried)	2 mg	Garlic (raw)	1.7 mg

- Iron is an essential mineral used to transport oxygen to all parts of our body.
- Deficiency—anemia, fatigue, weakness, organ failure.
- Black tea, calcium, peppermint tea, penny royal, cocoa, vervain, lime flower, milk, antacids chamomile, and herbal teas reduce iron absorption.

PROTEIN RICH DIET

Per 100 gm			
Food	Protein	Food	Protein
Almond nuts	21.1 g	Bacon	15.9 g
Baked beans	9.5 g	Bread (wholemeal)	11.0 g
Cheese	30.9 g	Chicken breast (skinless)	23.5 g
Cod fish	17.9 g	Eggs	12.5 g
Lamb (steak)	19.9 g	Lobster	26.41
Pasta	12.5 g	Peanut butter (crunchy)	24.9 g
Pizza (pepperoni)	11.4 g	Pork chops	19.3 g
Porridge oats	11.0 g	Prawns	17.0 g
Pumpkin seeds	28.8 g	Salmon fish fillets (boneless)	21.6 g
Soya beans	35.9 g	Sunflower seeds	23.4 g
Tuna fish (tinned)	26.3 g	Turkey breast (skinless)	22.3 g
Venison (deer meat)	30.21		

VITAMIN A RICH DIET

Per 100 gm			
Liver animal	1000 IU	Cod liver oil	500 IU
Paprika	52735 IU	Sweet potatoes	19218 IU
Raw carrots	16706 IU	Kale	15376 IU
Dark orange squash	11155 IU	Dried parsley	10184 IU
Red and green leaf lettuces	7492 IU	Dried apricots	3604 IU
Cantaloupe	3382 IU	Papaya	1094 IU
Mangoes	765 IU	Green peas	2100 IU
Tomatoes	833 IU	Whole milk	102 IU
Eggs (yolks)	538 IU		

- Vitamin A is an essential vitamin required for vision, gene transcription, boosting immune function, and great skin health.
- Fat-soluble vitamin.
- Deficiency—blindness.
- Overconsumption—jaundice, nausea, loss of appetite, irritability, vomiting, and hair loss.
- *Benefits*:
  - Protection from bacterial and viral infections
  - regulate the immune system
  - Lowers risk of many types of malignancy.

RICH IN VITAMIN B₁

Per 100 gm			
Yeast-thiamin	9.7 mg	Sesame butter	1.6 mg
Sunflower seeds	1.48 mg	Pine nuts	1.2 mg
Macadamia nuts	0.7 mg	Fish pompano	0.68 mg
Tuna fish	0.5 mg		

- Thiamin
- For maintaining cellular function
- Deficiency—beriberi and/or Wernicke-Korsakoff syndrome.

RICH IN VITAMIN B₂

Per 100 gm			
Yeast extract	14.3 mg	Lamb liver	4.6 mg
Dried chilies	2.26 mg	Paprika	1.74 mg
Chili powder	0.8 mg	Almonds	1.01 mg
Dry roasted soybeans	0.76 mg	Crude wheat bran	0.58 mg
Sesame seeds	0.47 mg	Sun-dried tomatoes	0.49 mg

- Riboflavin
- Water soluble vitamin
- Energy metabolism
- Deficiency—cracking and reddening of the lips, inflammation of the mouth, mouth ulcers, sore throat, and iron deficiency anemia.

RICH IN VITAMIN B₃

Per 100 gm			
Yeast	97 mg	Rice bran	34 mg
Wheat bran	13.6 mg	Paprika	15.3 mg
Peanuts	14.9 mg	Meat of chicken	12.4 mg
Bacon	11.6 mg	Sun-dried tomatoes	9.1 mg

- Niacin.
- Water soluble vitamin.
- Lowering cholesterol levels.
- Regulating blood sugar levels.
- Slow the progression of AIDS and increasing survival.
- Deficiency—pellagra (diarrhea, dermatitis, dementia), amnesia, delirium, irritability, poor concentration, anxiety, fatigue, restlessness, apathy, and depression.
- Overdose—skin rashes, dry skin, liver damage, elevated blood sugar, type II diabetes and increased risk of birth defects.

RICH IN VITAMIN B$_5$

Per 100 gm			
Chicken liver	8.3 mg	Rice bran	7.4 mg
Wheat bran	2.2 mg	Sunflower seeds	7.1 mg
Mushrooms	3.6 mg	Sun-dried tomatoes	2.1 mg
Avocados	1.5		

- Pantothenic acid.
- Water-soluble vitamin.
- Required by the body for cellular processes and optimal maintenance of fat.
- Deficiency—irritability, fatigue, apathy, numbness, paresthesia, and muscle cramps.

RICH IN VITAMIN B$_6$

Per 100 gm			
Rice bran	4.07 mg	Wheat bran	1.3 mg
Chili powder	3.67 mg	Raw garlic	1.235 mg
Liver	1.04 mg	Sunflower seeds	0.81 mg
Roasted sesame seeds	0.8 mg	Bananas	0.37 mg
Baked potato	0.31 mg	Oatmeal	0.29 mg
Cooked spinach	0.14 mg	Tomato juice	0.11 mg
Soybeans	0.06 mg		

- Pyridoxine, pyridoxal, pyridoxamine.
- Water-soluble vitamin
- Maintenance of red blood cell metabolism, the nervous system, the immune system.
- Deficiency—dermatitis, depression, confusion, convulsions, and anemia.

RICH IN FOLIC ACID

Per 100 gm			
Yeast extract	1010 µg	Dried spearmint	530 µg
Sunflower seeds	238 µg	Raw spinach	194 µg
Soybean sprouts	172 µg	Pea sprouts	144 µg
Chickpeas	172 µg	Mung beans	159 µg
Navy beans	140 µg	Asparagus	149 µg
Peanuts	145 µg	Oranges	30 µg
Papaya	38 µg	Bananas	20 µg

- Vitamin B_9.
- A water-soluble B vitamin.
- DNA synthesis and repair, cell division, and cell growth.
- Deficiency—anemia, slower development in children.
- Protects against heart disease, lower levels of homocysteine, boosts cardiovascular health and decreases risk of heart attacks.
- Decreases risk of breast, pancreatic, and colon malignancy.
- For absorption of vitamin B_{12}, folic acid is essential.
- In pregnant woman it prevents neural tube defect in babies.
- Decreased risk of Alzheimer's disease.

RICH IN VITAMIN B_{12}

Per 100 gm			
Eggs of whitefish	56.4 µg	Octopus	36 µg
Crab	11.5 µg	Lamb	3.71 µg
Swiss cheese	3.34 µg	Chicken eggs	1.95 µg
Yogurt (whole)	0.37 µg	Whole milk	0.44 µg
Goat milk and maize also contain vitamin B_{12}			

- Cobalamin.
- Vitamin B_{12} can only be manufactured by bacteria and can only be found naturally in animal products.
- Deficiency—anemia, fatigue, mania, and depression, permanent damage to the brain.

- *Useful*:
  - Protects against heart disease
  - Reduces malignancy risk
  - Protects against dementia
  - Alzheimer's disease.

VITAMIN C RICH DIET

Per 100 gm			
Green chillies	242.5 mg	Red chillies	144 mg
Guavas	228 mg	Simla mirch	184 mg
Green peppers	132 mg	Parsley	133 mg
Raw kale	120 mg	Broccoli	89 mg
Kiwi fruits	93 mg	Papaya	62 mg
Oranges	59 mg	Strawberries	59 mg
Acerola	1678 mg	Mangoes	28 mg
Tomatoes	23 mg	Banana peppers	83 mg
Coriander (dry)	567 mg		

- Vitamin C is an essential for the development and maintenance of scar tissue, blood vessels, and cartilage.
- A powerful antioxidant.
- Lowers malignancy risk.
- Lowers blood pressure.
- Reducing risk of heart attack.
- Boosting immune function.
- Helps in increased iron absorption.

VITAMIN D RICH DIET

Per 100 gm			
Cod liver oil	10001 IU	Fish	1628 IU
Oysters	320 IU	Caviar	232 IU
Eggs	37.0 IU		

- Vitamin D required for absorption of calcium, bone development, control of cell growth, neuromuscular functioning, proper immune functioning, and alleviation of inflammation.
- Deficiency—rickets, weakened immune system, increased malignancy risk, poor hair growth, and osteomalacia.
- Excess—risk of heart attack and kidney stones.

Per 100 gm			
Sunflower seeds	36.6 mg	Red chili powder	30 mg
Almonds provide	26.2 mg	Pine nuts	9.3 mg
Peanuts	6.9 mg	Basil and oregano	7.38 mg
Dried apricots	4.3 mg	Green olives	3.81 mg
Cooked spinach	3.5 mg	Wheat germ oil	149 mg
Soybean oil	8.2 mg		

VITAMIN E RICH DIET

- Vitamin E—fat-soluble vitamins
- Prevents oxidative stress to the body
- Protects against heart disease, malignancy and macular degeneration.
- Reduced risk of heart disease.
- Reduced malignancy risk.
- Help in type II diabetes.

VITAMIN K RICH FOODS

Per 100 gm			
Dried basil, dried sage	1715 µg	Kale	882 µg
Spring onions	207 µg	Brussel sprouts	194 µg
Broccoli	141 µg	Chili powder	106 µg
Asparagus	80 µg	Cabbage	76 µg
Pickled cucumber	77 µg	Prunes	60 µg
Okra	40 µg	Soybean oil	184 µg
Carrots	13 µg	Celery	29 µg
Jute	108 µg	Cloves	142 µg

- Vitamin K is an essential vitamin required for protein modification and blood clotting.
- Role in treating—osteoporosis and
  - Alzheimer's
  - Protects against malignancy
  - Prevents heart disease.

CALCIUM RICH DIET

Per 100 gm			
Dark leafy greens	120 mg	Cheese	961 mg
Yogurt	125 mg	Chinese cabbage	105 mg
Soy	350 mg	Okra	77 mg
Broccoli	47 mg	Green snap beans	37 mg
Almonds	264 mg	Cheese	1376 mg
Milk	113 mg	Fish	74 mg
Garlic	181 mg		

Calcium is necessary for the growth and maintenance of strong teeth and bones, nerve signaling, muscle contraction, and secretion of certain hormones and enzymes.

- Deficiency—numbness in fingers and toes, muscle cramps, convulsions, lethargy, loss of appetite, and abnormal heart rhythms, bone health and osteoporosis.

IODINE RICH DIET

Dried seaweed	4.5 mg in 1/4 ounce
Iodized salt fortified	77 µg/gram
Baked potato with peel	60 µg/1 medium
Milk	56 µg/cup
Fish sticks	35 µg/2 sticks
Egg boiled	12 µg/1 egg

- Iodine is a chemical element essential for the production of thyroid hormones that regulate growth and metabolism.
- Deficient—Cretinism, mental slowness, high cholesterol, lethargy, fatigue, depression, weight gain and goiter.

POTASSIUM RICH FOOD

Per 100 gm			
White beans	561 mg	Dark leafy greens (spinach)	558 mg
Baked potatoes	535 mg	Dried apricots	1162 mg
Bananas	358 mg	Mushrooms (white)	396 mg
Avocados	485 mg	Fish (salmon)	628 mg
Yogurt (plain, skim/non-fat)	255 mg	Baked acorn squash	437 mg
Dried herbs (parsley, chervil, corriander, basil, dill)	4740 mg	Cocoa powder and dark chocolate	2509 mg
Dry roasted soybeans	1364 mg	Rice bran	1485 mg
Sunflower seeds	850 mg	Coconut water	250 mg
Orange juice	200 mg		
Dates	696 mg (20% DV)		

- Potassium is an essential nutrient used to maintain fluid and electrolyte balance in the body.

- Deficiency—fatigue, irritability, and hypertension, osteoporosis.

Rice bran	1677 mg	Oat	690 mg/cup
Roasted pumpkin and squash seeds	1172 mg	Sunflower seeds	1158 mg
Wheat germ	1146 mg	Cheese	807 mg
Sesame seeds	774 mg	Brazil nuts	725 mg
Roasted soybeans	649 mg	Flax seeds	642 mg
Bacon	591 mg	Poppy seeds	849 mg

PHOSPHORUS RICH DIET

- Phosphorus is an essential nutrient required for proper cell functioning, regulation of calcium, strong bones and teeth.

- Deficiency—lowered appetite, anemia, muscle pain, rickets, numbness, and a weakened immune system.

ZINC RICH DIET

Oysters	16–182 mg/100 g	Toasted wheat germ	17 mg/100 g
Veal liver	12 mg/100 g	Rosted beef	10 mg/100 g
Pumpkin and squash seeds	10 mg/100 g	Dried watermelon seeds	10 mg/100 g
Baking chocolate	9.6 mg/100 g	Cocoa powder	6.8 mg/100 g
Lamb	4.2–8.7 mg/100 g	Peanuts	6.6 mg/100 g
Crab	7.6 mg/100 g	Chicken leg	2.9 mg/100 g
Dry roasted cashews	5.6 mg/100 g	Almonds	3.5 mg/100 g
Milk	0.4 mg/100 g		

- Zinc is an essential mineral required by the body for maintaining a sense of smell, keeping a healthy immune system, building proteins, triggering enzymes and creating DNA.
- Deficiency—stunted growth, diarrhea, impotence, hair loss, eye and skin lesions, impaired appetite, and depressed immunity.
- Excess—nausea, vomiting, loss of appetite, abdominal cramps, diarrhea, and headaches disrupt absorption of copper and iron in the long term.

CHOLESTEROL RICH DIET

Per 100 gm			
Yolks of eggs	1234 mg	Whole egg	212 mg
Fish	588 mg	Liver (meat)	564 mg
Butter	215 mg/packs	Cheeses	123 mg
Shellfish	105 mg	Biscuits, burgers and sandwiches	235 mg
Ice cream	92 mg	Whole milk	10 mg

- Cholesterol is a steroid lipid (fat) found in the blood of all animals and is necessary for proper functioning of our cell membranes and production of hormones.
- Cholesterol is only found in animal food products.
- Excessive consumption of cholesterol increases the risk of heart disease and stroke.

SATURATED FAT RICH DIET

Per 100 gm			
Palm and/or coconut oil	86.5 g	Dried unsweetened coconut	57 gm
Raw coconut meat	27 gm	Butter	51 gm
Animal fats	35–45 gm	Oat cheese	24 gm

- Saturated fat has long been associated with increased risk of heart disease, stroke, and malignancy.

FIBER RICH DIET

Per 100 gm			
Corn, wheat, rice, oat	79 g	Seeds (flax seeds, sesame, sunflower, pumpkin)	27 g
Cocoa powder and dark chocolate	33 g	Nuts (almonds, hazel—nuts, pine nuts, pistachios, pecans)	12 g
Beans	11 g	Sun dried tomatoes	12 g
Popcorn	15 g	Baked potato	2 g
Oranges	2 g	Figs (Dried)	9.8 g
Apricots (Dried)	7.3 g	Coconut (Dried)	16.3 g
Avocados	7 g	Dates	6.7 g
Guavas	5.4 g	Bran	79 g
Cauliflower & Broccoli	2.4 g	Cabbage	3 g
Raspberries	7 g	Celery	2 g
Beans (Kidney)	6 g		

CARBOHYDRATES RICH DIET

Dehydrated apple, prunes, bananas	Dried peaches and apricots
Raisins	Dates
Cookies and cakes	Flours
Jams	Potato
French fries	

- Play a critical role in the proper functioning of the immune system, fertilization, pathogenesis, blood clotting, and human development.

MANGANESE RICH DIET

Cloves	30 mg/100 gm	Toasted wheat germ	20 mg
Wheat bran provides	6.7 mg per cup	Rice bran provides	16.8 mg/cup
Oat bran provides	2.1 mg/cup	Hazelnuts	12.7 mg/100 gm
Pine nuts	2.5 mg/ounce	Pecans	1.3 mg/ounce
Shellfish	6.8 mg/100 gm	Unsweetened baking chocolate	4.2 mg/100 g
Cocoa powder	3.8 mg/100 gm	Pumpkin and squash seeds	0.5 mg/100 gm
Chili powder	2.2 mg/100 gm	Roasted soybeans	2.2 mg/100 gm
Sunflower seeds	2.11 mg/100 gm		

- Manganese is required by the body for proper enzyme functioning, nutrient absorption, wound healing, and bone development.
- Manganese deficiency leads to joint pain and fertility problems.

Benefits

- *Antioxidant protection*: Manganese superoxide dismutase is antioxidant in the mitochondria.
- Osteoporosis protection
- Prevention of epileptic seizures
- Prevention of alopecia

HIGHEST IN SODIUM

Table salt	100 grams of table salt provides 38,000 mg
Baking soda	One teaspoon of baking soda provides 1368 mg of sodium
Baking powder	One teaspoon of baking powder contains 530 mg
Soy sauce	One teaspoon contains 335 mg
Yeast extract	One teaspoon providing 216 mg
Bacon	One slice of bacon (8 grams) contains 194 mg of sodium
Beef jerky	1 large piece (20 g) contains 443 mg of sodium
Sun dried tomatoes	100 grams provide 2095 mg of sodium
Salt water crab	100 grams provides 1072 mg of sodium

- Sodium is an essential nutrient required for the body for maintaining levels of fluids and for providing channels of nerve signaling.

- Deficiency of sodium occurs after excessive vomiting or diarrhea, in athletes who intake excessive amounts of water, or in people who regularly fast on juice and water.
- Overconsumption of sodium is far more common and can lead to high blood pressure, increased risk of heart attack and stroke.

FOODS HIGH IN POTASSIUM

Winter squash	(1 cup 1 gm)	Dried apricots	(1/2 cup 0.9 gm)
Baked potato	(1 large 0.9 g)	Swiss chard	(960 mg per 1 cup)
Avocado	(874 mg per cup)	Spinach	(838 mg per cup)
Crimini mushrooms	(635 mg in 5 ounces)	Broccoli	(505 mg per cup)
Brussels sprouts	(494 mg per cup)	Celery	(344 mg per cup)

IRON RICH VEGETABLES

	(mg/1 cup)		
Soybeans	8.84	Soybeans	4.50
Spinach boiled	6.43	Tomatoes	5.00
Parsley raw	4.00	Swiss Chard	3.96
Pumpkin	3.41	Turnip greens	3.18
Beets	3.09	Dandelion greens	1.89
Kale	1.22	Broccoli raw	0.64

PROTEIN RICH VEGETABLES

	(1 cup)		
Alfalfa seeds	1.32	Corn	4.51
Artichokes	4.18	Cowpeas	5.23
Asparagus	5.31	Dandelion greens	2.1
Beans	12.17	Kidney beans	15.35
Beet greens	3.7	Lentils	17.86
Beets	2.86	Lima beans	14.66
Broccoli	2.62	Mung beans	3.16
Cabbage	1.01	Mushrooms	3.39
Carrots	1.13	Mustard greens	3.16
Cauliflower	1.98	Navy beans	15.83
Celery	1.25	Okra	3.83

HIGH CALCIUM FOODS

Per 100 gm			
Milk	290 to 300 mg	Alfalfa sprouts	11 mg
Yogurt	240 to 400 mg	Beets	44 mg
Egg	55 mg	Carrot	42 mg/1 cup
Cottage cheese	80 to 100 mg	Celery	41 mg/1 cup
Ice cream	80–100 mg	Cauliflower	10 mg/1 cup
Broccoli	180 mg/cup	Cucumber	17 mg/1 cup
Kale cabbage	90–100 mg ½ cup	Tomatoes	94 mg/1 cup
Okra-okra	70 mg ½ cup	Green beans	55 mg
Turnip greens	100–125 mg ½ cup	Potatoes	26 mg/1 cup
Spinach	300 mg/cup	Milk	290–300 mg
Yogurt	240–400 mg		

HEALTHIEST VEGETABLES

Broccoli	Mustard and turnip greens
Cauliflower	Tomatoes
Brussels sprouts	Leeks
Green and red cabbage	Onions
Carrots	Shallots
Kale	Scallions
Spinach	Garlic
Swiss chard	Sweet potatoes and yams
Collard greens	Bell peppers
The herb parsley	Summer and winter squash
Red and green lettuce	Mustard and turnip greens

HEALTHIEST FRUIT

Apples	Apricots
Bananas	Berries
Cantaloupes	Cherries
Citrus fruits: Oranges, lemons and limes	Kiwi fruit
Papayas	Red grapes

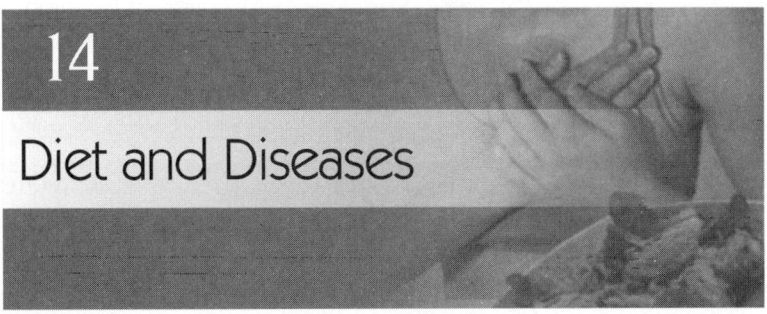

14

Diet and Diseases

1. Nephrotic Syndrome

- A balanced diet adequate in both energy and protein (1–2 gm per kilogram body weight).
- A high calorie diet.
- Low fat content because of high serum triglycerides levels of these patients.
- Low sodium levels in the diet.
- Salt should be restricted.

Foodstuffs rich in protein: A cow's milk, skimmed milk, eggs, fish, dry fish, chicken, lean meat, paneer made from cow's milk, cheese, sprouts, pulses and legumes such as tur dal, moong dal, rajmah, chana, lentils.

Foodstuffs high in sodium: Baking soda, salt, ajinomoto, salted wafers, popcorns, salted biscuits, papads. All varieties, salted pickles, chutneys, curry powder, soft drinks containing sodium benzoate, vakery products, bread, biscuits, nuts such as salted cashew nuts, pistachio, walnuts, peanuts, sea food, chicken, dry fish, bournvita, chocolate drinks, horlicks, milk and curds, pulses and legumes—all varieties. Vegetables such as—cauliflower, snake gourd, beetroot, carrot, coriander leaves, fenugreek (methi) leaves, lettuce, spinach (palak), amaranth, radish.

2. Diabetes Mellitus

- Meals and snacks should be eaten at regular intervals.
- Physical activity is very important part of child's day.

- Child should have an extra snack.
- Sugary drink or sweet in case the child's blood glucose level drops to low.
- May need to eat some starchy food, such as sandwich depending on timing of activity and level of exercise taken.
- Artificial sweeteners does not contain sugar, therefore, they will not raise blood glucose level.
- Sweeteners can be used instead of sugar when making milkshakes, khir, tea, coffee, and milk.

3. Chronic Renal Failure

- Provide adequate calories
- Regulate the protein content of the diet
- Regulate sodium, potassium and fluid intake
- Restrict phosphate and supplement the diet with calcium, iron, trace minerals, ascorbic acid and the B-complex vitamins.
- Sodium restriction is necessary

  Foodstuffs high in sodium: Baking soda, salt, ajinomoto, salted wafers, popcorns, salted biscuits, papads—all varieties, salted pickles, chutneys, curry powder, soft drinks containing sodium benzoate, bakery products, bread, biscuits, nuts such as salted cashew nuts, pistachio, walnuts, peanuts, sea food, chicken, dry fish, bournvita, chocolate drinks, horlicks, milk and curds, pulses and legumes—all varieties. Vegetables such as—cauliflower, snake gourd, beetroot, carrot, coriander leaves, fenugreek(methi) leaves, lettuce, spinach (palak), amaranth, radish.

- Restricted potassium in the diet.

  Foods low in potassium: Rice, vegetables such as cucumber, ridge gourd (turai), snake gourd (padwal), tinda, broad beans, beetroot, fenugreek leaves (methi), green mango, pink radish, bottle gourd (dudhi) guava, papaya, pear, tea.

4. Kidney Stones

Calcium oxalate stones:

- Fluid intake increased to 3000 ml/day or more depending on the tolerance of the patient.

- Avoid a high protein diet.
- *Calcium restriction*: Cereals such as ragi, whole bengal, gram (chana), moth beans (matki), rajmah, soya beans, horse gram (kuleeth). All green leafy vegetables.
- *Oxalate restriction*: Horsegram (kuleeth), kesari dal, almonds, cashew nuts, gingelly seeds, ripe chillies, amla, wood apple, cocoa, coffee, tea, green leafy vegetables such as amaranth, curry leaves, drumstick leaves, mustard leaves, neem leaves, colocasia leaves, dry lotus stem, green plantain, dry coconut, gingelly seeds (til), mustard seeds, asafoetida (hing), dry cloves, coriander and cumin seeds, poppy seeds.
- Avoid taking vitamin, mineral supplements.
- Avoid too much vitamin C and calcium containing antacids.
- Avoid vegetables and fruits containing seeds such as tomatoes, lady finger, brinjal, capsicum, watermelon, guava, etc.

Uric acid stones: Avoid purine rich foods like organ meats such as kidney, liver, pancreas, brain, sweet breads and meat extracts.

5. Hepatitis

- A high caloric diet
- *Carbohydrate*: An intake of 6–8 gm/kg carbohydrate ensures adequate glycogen reserves needed for the maintenance of liver function for protection against further injury to the liver and for its protein sparing action.
- *Protein*: An intake of 1 ½ to 2 grams protein per kg of body weight is recommended to overcome negative nitrogen balance to promote regeneration of parenchymal cell, and to prevent fatty infiltration of the liver.
- *Fat*: Diets restricted in fats are not necessary in the majority of patients with hepatitis. If there is anorexia, fats may cause nausea and should be limited to amounts tolerated by the patient.
- Foods in liquid or soft; consistency are preferable.

6. Cancer

- Children with cancer have increased calories and protein needs.
- Protein is needed for growth and to help the body repair itself.
- Foods should be high in fat.
- Kheer, ice cream, milk shake, vegetables, dhal, soups, coffee, tea.
- Full fat milk (buffalo's milk), cream (malai).
- Cheese, dahi, ghee, eggs, honey sugar, condensed milk, nuts, beans and legumes (dal).

7. Protein Energy Malnutrition

- Milk + sugar
- Egg
- Ragi porridge, wheat flour porridge or rava porridge
- Khichdi with mashed vegetables, upma
- Rice + dal
- Fruit juice
- Vegetable soup
- One banana
- Continue breast-milk feeding
- Use clean environment and with boiled water whenever required.

8. Cardiovascular Diseases

Eat more in quantity: Raw nuts, olive oil, fish oils, flax seeds, or avocados, colorful fruits and vegetables, cereals, breads, legumes, fish and shellfish, poultry and egg white.

Eat less: Whole-fat dairy or red meat, packaged foods (high in sodium), white or egg breads, granola-type cereals, refined pastas or rice, red meat, bacon, sausage, fried chicken, egg yolks, potato chips.

Best foods for lowering cholesterol are oatmeal, fish, walnuts and olive oil.

9. Wilson Disease

- Drinking water may contain elevated levels of copper. Copper content of water should be less than 0.1 ppm.
- Food labels to see if they contain copper.
- Vitamins are high in copper and should be avoided.
- Copper cooking utensils can leave trace amounts in food and should not be used.
- *Avoid high copper foods*: Lamb, pork, quail, duck, goose, shellfish, nuts and seeds, mushrooms, raisins, dates, prunes, avocado, dried beans, soya beans, lima beans, baked beans, garbanzo beans, pinto beans, dried peas, lentils, millet, barley, wheat germ.

10. Thalassemia

- Iron overload problem due to regular blood transfusion.
- Avoid iron rich diet like dried herbs, cocoa powder and chocolate, liver of animals (duck, chicken, pork, lamb, turkey and beef), clams, oysters and mussels, roasted pumpkin and squash seeds, sesame butter and seeds, sun dried tomatoes, sunflower seeds, dried apricots, kidney bean, soya bean, chicken leg.
- *Take antioxidant*: Green tea, corn, kale, plums, berries, peaches, peppers, spinach, cherries, tomatoes, cantaloupe.

15

Nutrition Related Organizations

UNICEF

UNICEF is committed to scaling up and sustaining coverage of its current high-impact nutrition interventions in the programme areas of:
- Infant and young child feeding
- Micronutrients
- Nutrition security in emergencies
- Nutrition and HIV/AIDS
- Providing nutrition security and nutrition in emergencies
- Monitoring infant growth rates
- Infant and child feeding and care
- Delivering vital micronutrients.

NUTRITION SOCIETY OF INDIA

- It was established in 1967.
- This is an organization dedicated to keep abreast of the latest developments in the basic and applied aspects of science of nutrition. It has the following aims related to nutrition:
  - To be the representative organization of nutrition professionals from Mumbai and India.
  - To exchange views in nutrition and allied sciences through meetings, symposia seminars and workshops.
  - To disseminate knowledge in nutrition to the common man through meetings, symposia, seminars and workshops organized by the members.

NATIONAL INSTITUTE OF NUTRITION, HYDERABAD, INDIA

- Founded by Sir Robert McCarrison in the year 1918 at the Pasteur Institute, Connor, Tamil Nadu.
- In 1928 it emerged as full-fledged "Nutrition Research Laboratories" Dr McCarrison was as its first Director.
- In 1958, it was shifted to Hyderabad.
- In 1969, it was renamed as National Institute of Nutrition.
- It has attained global recognition for its pioneering studies on various aspects of nutrition research, with special reference to protein energy malnutrition.

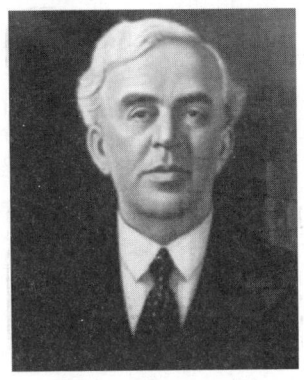

Sir Robert McCarrison—the founder

Objectives

- To identify various dietary and nutrition problems prevalent among different segments of the population in the country.
- To continuously monitor diet and nutrition situation of the country.
- To evolve effective methods of management and prevention of nutritional problems.

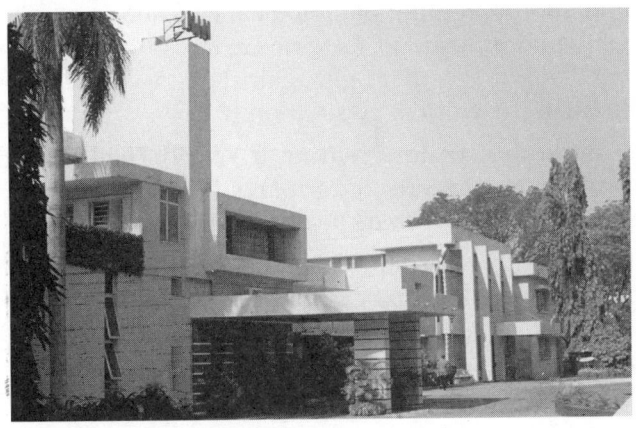

- To conduct operational research connected with planning and implementation of National Nutrition Programmes.
- To dovetail nutrition research with other health programmes of the government.
- Human resource development in the field of nutrition.

WORLD HEALTH NUTRITION ORGANIZATION

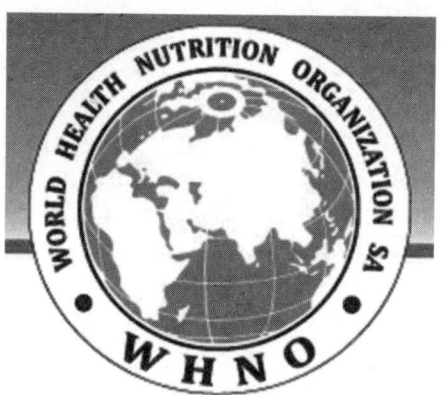

World Health Nutrition Organization is an independent non-government and nonpolitical organization headquarter in Switzerland.

Main objective is educating people about healthy and proper nutrition and preventing pathological conditions and diseases caused by poor nutrition. Also aims to stress the importance of an immediate and regular fight against overweight and obesity that threaten the world's population.

The main motive for creating a World Health Nutrition Organization is a sincere concern about the rate of obesity and its negative effect on people's health and the quality of their lives.

World Health Nutrition Organization has regional offices throughout the world that carry out its mission and goals.

One of the main tasks of these offices is to organize various events to call attention to the principles of healthy eating habits and proper nutrition.

Aims

- Prevention of extra weight
- Availability of ecologically pure food
- Body detox
- Minimize the effects of aging by means of correctly selected food.
- Promotion of healthy and correct nutrition
- Development and support of programs aimed to prolong and improve the quality of people's lives by improving the quality of their nutrition
- Development and support of programs that help prevent diseases caused by improper nutrition
- Development and support of events and measures that fight overweight and obesity
- Incorporation of scientific, organizational, manufacturing, and financial resources that combat improper nutrition, overweight, and obesity
- Development of new technologies of cooking food products that seek to reduce the negative effect of overweight and obesity
- Implementation and support of various programs promoting ecological products
- Development, support, and certification of healthy nutrition programs.

WORLD FOOD DAY

- It is celebrated on 16 October in honor of the date of the founding of the Food and Agriculture Organization of the United Nations in 1945.
- Dr Pal Romany, Hungarian Minister of Agriculture and Food, was the founder member of this.
- Its office is at Washington, DC.
- It is celebrated every year in more than 150 countries, raising awareness of the nutrition behind poverty and hunger.

- The World Food Day theme for 2012 was "Agricultural cooperatives—key to feeding the world".

WORLD NUTRITION DAY

1st September

REFERENCES

1. *Nutrition*: Wikipedia, the free encyclopedia.

Index